Strength Training Today
Second Edition

Bob O'Connor

Jerry Simmons
Strength and Conditioning Coach
Carolina Panthers

Pat O'Shea
Professor Emeritus of Physical Education
Oregon State University

Series Editor
Bob O'Connor, Ed. D.

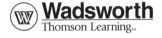

Wadsworth
Thomson Learning™

Australia • Canada • • Mexico • Singapore • Spain • United Kingdom • United States

Publisher: Peter Marshall
Editorial Assistant: Keynia Johnson
Project Editor: Matt Stevens
Print Buyer: April Reynolds
Permissions Editor: Joohee Lee
Production: Fritz/Brett Associates Inc.
Interior and Cover Designer: Harry Voigt Graphic Design

Copyeditor: Susan Defosset
Illustrator: Kevin Somerville
Cover Image: © Carl Vanderschuit/
    FPG International LLC
Compositor: Pat Rogondino
Printer/Binder: Webcom Ltd.
Photography: David Hanover, Gehrhard Pagels,
    Kristine Krangler

Printed in Canada

1   2   3   4   5   6   7   03   02   01   00   99

Library of Congress Cataloging-in-Publication Data
O'Connor, Robert, 1932–
    Strength training today / Bob O'Connor, Jerry Simmons,
Pat O'Shea.—2nd ed.
        p. cm.
    Rev. ed. of: Weight training today. 1989.
    Includes bibliographical references ( ) and index.
    ISBN 0-534-35837-3
    1. Weight training. I. Simmons, Jerry. II. O'Shea, Pat, 1930–
III. O'Connor, Robert, 1932– Weight training today. IV. Title.

GV546.036 2000
613.7'13—dc21   99-047559

♺ This book is printed on acid-free recycled paper.

For more information, contact

Wadsworth/Thomson Learning
10 Davis Drive
Belmont, CA 94002-3098
USA
www.wadsworth.com

International Headquarters
Thomson Learning
290 Harbor Drive, 2nd Floor
Stamford, CT 06902-7477
USA

UK/Europe/Middle East/South Africa
Thomson Learning
Berkshire House
168-173 High Holborn
London WC1V 7AA
United Kingdom

Asia
Thomson Learning
60 Albert Street #15-01
Albert Complex
Singapore 189969

Canada
Nelson/Thomson Learning
1120 Birchmount Road
Scarborough, Ontario M1K 5G4
Canada

Contents

Preface vii

1 Introduction to Strength Training 1
History of Strength Training 2
Reasons for Strength Training 2
Who Can Profit from Strength Training 3
Proper Attire 3
    Checklist for Workout Attire 4
Medical Clearance 4
Summary 4

2 How to Get What You Want from Strength Training 5
Aspects of General Fitness 6
Planning Your Strength-Training Program 6
    Checklist for Terms Commonly Used 7
General Body Conditioning 7
Developing Strength 7
Developing Muscle Hypertrophy 8
    Checklist for Developing Muscle Hypertrophy 9
Hormonal Factors 10
Developing Muscular Endurance 10
Developing Power and Speed 11
Plyometrics 11
Developing Flexibility 12
Developing Better Posture 12
Becoming a More Effective Athlete 13
Rehabilitating Muscles After Injury 13
Body Contouring 13
Body Measurements 14
Body Weight 14
Measuring Body Fat 14
    Girth Measurements 15
Muscle Balance 17
Cardiovascular/Cardiorespiratory Endurance 17
Summary 17

3 The Physiology and Biomechanics of Strength Training 19
Muscles 20
    Checklist for Understanding Muscle Fiber 21
Lever Action 21
Types of Muscular Contractions 22
Types of Exercises 23
Types of Resistance 23
    Checklist for Buying Home Exercise Equipment 25
Body Positions 26
Joint Actions 26
Isolating a Muscle 26
Doing a Coordinated Movement 26
Proper Breathing 27
    Checklist for Breathing During a Normal Strength Workout 27
    Checklist for Breathing in Weight-Lifting Competition 28

Warm-Up 28
   Checklist for Warm-Up 29
Soreness 29
Summary 29

4   Choosing Your Workout Schedule 31
Exercise Order 32
Workout for Strength 32
Priority System 32
   Cyclic System 33
   Pyramid System 33
   Reverse Pyramid System 33
Workout for Muscle Bulk 33
   Split Routines 34
   Super Sets 34
Workout for General Body Conditioning 34
   The Karvonen Formula 35
Rest Between Sets 36
Rest Between Workouts 36
Periodization 36
Recording Your Progress 37
   Checklist for Recording Your Progress 38
   Checklist for Workouts 39
Summary 41

5   The Mental Approach to Strength Training 43
Setting Goals 44
The Mental Benefits of Strength Training 44
Imagery 45
   Checklist for Mental Imagery 45
Relaxation 46
Concentration 46
Mental Training Works 46
Rehearse Success 47
Summary 47

6   Flexibility Exercises 49
Shoulder and Chest 50
Groin 51
Lower Back and Hamstrings 51
Trunk 52
Thigh and Groin 53
Calf 54
Triceps 54
New Research on Stretching 54
   Checklist for Workout Progression 56
Summary 56

7   Single-Joint (Isolation) Exercises 57
Determining the Desired Outcome 58
Selecting the Exercises 58
Selecting the Equipment 58
Isolating the Joint Action 60
   1. Neck 60
   2. Shoulders 62

3. Chest 67
4. Upper Back 70
5. Abdominals 74
Checklist for Abdominal Exercises 76
6. Lower Back 77
7. Hip Flexors 79
8. Knee Extensors (Leg Extension) 82
9. Hip (Thigh) Extensors 83
10. Knee Flexors (Leg Curls) 85
11. Ankle Plantar Flexion 87
12. Other Ankle Exercises 89
13. Arm (Elbow) Flexion 91
14. Arm (Elbow) Extension (Triceps Extension) 94
15. Wrist Flexion (Front of Forearms) 97
16. Wrist Extension (Back of Forearms) 99
17. Hip Abduction 100
18. Hip Adduction 102
Summary 104

8 Multiple-Joint Exercises 105
Multiple-Joint Exercises 106
19. Bench Press 106
Checklist for Safety 107
20. Incline Bench Press 108
21. Overhead (Military, or Shoulder) Barbell Press 108
Checklist for Loading and Unloading a Barbell 111
22. Lat Pull-Downs and Chin-Ups on a High Bar 111
23. Squat (Leg Press) 112
24. Lunge 115
25. Upright Row 115
26. Bent Row 116
27. Power Clean 116
28. Power Snatch 119
Checklist for the Snatch 119
Summary 120

9 Exercises for Special Interests—Posture and Sports 121
Exercises for Better Posture 122
Pot Belly 122
Round Shoulders 123
Checklist for Posture 124
Sagging Chest 124
Forward Head 124
Overall Posture 124
Exercises for Better Athletic Performance 125
The General Strength Program 125
The Specific Programs 125
Checklist for the Clean and Jerk 128
Checklist for General Muscle Strength 129
Cardiovascular Endurance 129
Considerations for the Female Athlete 130
Summary 130

10 Nutrition for Better Conditioning 131
Nutrition 132

Protein 133
Fats 135
Carbohydrates 137
Fiber 138
Vitamins 138
Checklist for Effective Eating 139
Minerals 139
Phytochemicals 141
Water 142
Summary 143

11   **Sensible Eating and Weight Management 145**
Important Considerations in Selecting Your Diet 146
Beverages 149
Food Additives 151
Vegetarianism 151
Smart Shopping 152
Eating and Overeating 152
    Should You Lose Weight? 153
How to Lose Weight 153
Calories Burned with Various Activities 155
Eating Disorders 155
Summary 157
Self-Test 157
Bulimia Self-Test 158
Where to Go for Help 158

12   **Ergogenics 161**
Aids to Building Muscle 162
    Nutrition Supplements 162
    Steroids 163
Increasing Anaerobic Capacity 164
Fluid and Carbohydrate Replacement 165
Muscle Recovery and Pain Reduction 167
Endurance Enhancement 167
Summary 167

13   **Strength-Training Injuries 169**
Strains and Sprains 170
Back Injuries 170
Knee Injuries 171
Arthritis and Joint-Wearing Injuries 171
High Blood Pressure 171
Blackouts 171
Other Injuries 172
Injury Prevention 172
Summary 172

APPENDICES 173
A: Essential Information on Vitamins and Minerals 173
B: Sources of Additional Information (Organizations and Publications) 181
C: Power Lifting: Types of Lifts 183
D: Weight Record Chart 184

Glossary of Strength-Training Terms 185

Index 189

Preface

This is a book for interested students and other people who want to learn more about strength training. It is not a book for those who will make a profession of teaching and training, although it may well be of benefit to such people.

This book explains the basic principles of modern scientific strength training. No other sport or method of exercise has changed as much in the last few decades. Beginning from the lore of early strong men about how they gained their strength, weight training has since become the most scientific area of physical education. Its popularity has increased, too, as the myths about muscleboundness have faded and people have come to realize that strength and fitness are appropriate to people of both sexes and every age group.

The growing emphasis on science has led to many new theories on how muscles contract, how fuels are stored in the muscles, how many repetitions are best for the development of strength, and so on. As new findings have been added to the science of weight training, many older ideas have been proven scientifically inaccurate. For this reason, the reader may find that current thinking is quite different from what was "known" in the past.

It is our sincere belief that by improving your knowledge of the principles of strength training, you will be able to increase the efficiency of your workout programs.

Acknowledgments

The development of this text could not have progressed without the helpful criticism and suggestions from our colleagues. We gratefully acknowledge the reviewers of this edition: Stephen Bronzan, University of California at Davis; Kelly Cordes, University of Montana; Andrew P. Jenkins, Central Washington University; George Katsikas; Lillian Pelios; and Kristopher Williams, University of Wisconsin at Oshkosh. We would also like to acknowledge our colleagues who reviewed the first edition: Bernard V. Buck, Shoreline Community College, Seattle; John Burgess, Suffolk Community College; Lynn Harbertson, Portland Community College; D. J. LeRoy, University of Wisconsin, Stevens Point; Renata Maiorino, University of Missouri, Columbia; Bill Mortiz, Moraine Valley Community College, Illinois; Maureen Murphy, Pima Community College, Tucson; Jay Roelen, Saddleback College, Mission Viejo; Dave Van Halanger, Florida State University, Tallahassee; Tom Ward, University of Texas at Austin; Owen J. Wilkinson, Ohio University, Athens.

We are also grateful to Christine Wells for her contributions to the nutrition and diet chapters. Thanks also to David Hanover, Gerhard Pagels, and Kristine Kranzler for their excellent photography, and to the models, Turid Agnete Teiger, Lars Tveter, and Quincy Douglas.

Bob O'Connor
Jerry Simmons
Pat O'Shea

Wadsworth's Physical Education Series

Aerobics Today, by Carole Casten and Peg Jordan

Aqua Aerobics Today, by Carol Casten

Badminton Today, by Tariq Wadood and Karlyne Tan

Golf Today, 2nd edition, by J. C. Snead and John L. Johnson

Jazz Dance Today, by Lorraine Person Kriegel and Kim Chandler-Vaccaro

Racquetball Today, by Lynn Adams and Erwin Goldbloom

Strength Training Today, 2nd edition, by Bob O'Connor, Jerry Simmons, and Pat O'Shea

Swimming and Aquatics Today, by Ron Ballatore, William Miller, and Bob O'Connor

Tennis Today, 2nd edition, by Glenn Bassett, William Otta, and Christine Shelton

Volleyball Today, 2nd edition, by Marv Dunphy and Rod Wilde

The Series Editor for Wadsworth's Physical Education Series

Dr. Bob O'Connor received his B.S. and M.S. degrees in physical education from UCLA and his doctorate from U.S.C. His 40-year teaching experience includes instruction in physical education courses for tennis, weight training, volleyball, badminton, swimming, and various team sports, as well as classes in teaching methods. Internationally, Dr. O'Connor has been an advisor to several Olympic programs in weight training and swimming. He was among the first to popularize strength training for all athletic events. Dr. O'Connor has written extensively in the fields of physical education and health.

1 *Introduction to Strength Training*

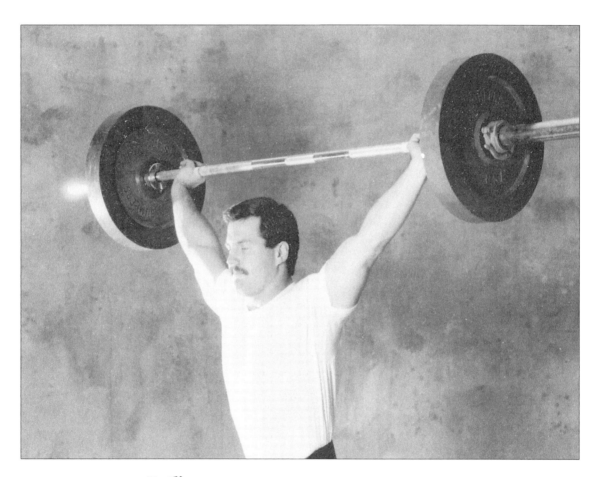

Outline

History of Strength Training
Reasons for Strength Training
Who Can Profit from Strength Training
Proper Attire
Checklist for Workout Attire
Medical Clearance
Summary

History of Strength Training

For thousands of years people have lifted weights to gain strength. In ancient Greece there is evidence that a man named Eumastas lifted a rock weighing over half a ton. You may have heard of an ancient Greek named Milo who lifted a calf every day. As the calf grew into a cow, Milo grew stronger and stronger. He showed off his strength by carrying the four-year-old cow the full length of the Olympic stadium—over 200 yards. This story illustrates the principle of *progressive resistance exercise* in which the muscles are overloaded to make them adapt by becoming stronger.

The Greeks used dumbbell-like weights called *halteres* 1,800 years ago, and weight training was popular with both men and women in ancient Rome. So, training with weights for strength and fitness is not a recent phenomenon. In fact, weight-lifting competition has been in the modern Olympic Games since they were reborn in 1896. Feats of strength that have delighted onlookers included Louis Cyr's lifting of 4,300 pounds from the floor in 1885 and, eight years later, noted strong woman Minervia's lifting of a platform holding 23 men—a weight of 3,564 pounds.

Our modern scientific strength training got its start after World War II, when Dr. Thomas DeLorme verified empirically that progressive resistance exercise could aid recovery of strength in wounded arms and legs. His studies made weight training scientifically and educationally respectable, finally banishing the idea that it leads to muscleboundness.

Reasons for Strength Training

Today people lift weights for a variety of reasons, which can be categorized as follows:

1. To compete in two Olympic weight lifts—the snatch and the clean and jerk (Olympic lifting)
2. To compete in the squat, bench press, and the dead lift (power lifting)
3. To contour the body to perceived ideal proportions (bodybuilding), as for the Mr. America or Miss America type of competition, or for beauty contests
4. To become more proficient in a sport by working on specific strength programs
5. To improve general fitness
6. To rehabilitate injured muscles
7. To prevent osteoporosis (soft bones)
8. To complete a physical education program that requires strength training classes
9. To develop a better self-concept by contouring the body to be closer to one's ideal

The average man or woman working with weights in a physical education class, a gym, or at home is generally working to gain some strength, but mainly to look and feel better. No matter what one's age, strength training is a valuable type of exercise. It positively affects several body systems, including muscular, endocrine, skeletal, metabolic, immune, neural, and respiratory.[1]

Who Can Profit from Strength Training

People of all ages and both sexes can profit from strength training. Younger people can develop bodies that are more efficient and generally considered to be more desirable—whether through muscle toning, reduced body fat, or larger muscles.

Older people, particularly women, can often reverse the process of osteoporosis that comes with aging if calcium has been insufficient in the diet and weight-bearing exercise has been lacking. Strength training can greatly reduce the number of broken bones that are suffered by the elderly. In addition, strengthened muscles help counteract the loss of muscle fibers that occurs as people age. Between the ages of 25 and 50, the number of muscle fibers drops by 5 to 10 percent; the number is reduced even more—by 25 to 30 percent—by age 80.[2]

Psychologists and sociologists who study the body are recognizing the essential relationship between satisfaction with one's body and self-esteem. So a well-conditioned body can help promote psychological well-being. Traditionally, the average female body has been far less conditioned than the average male body, but the acceptance of sport and exercise for women has allowed a gender equality in the physical realm.

People who run or play sports can reduce their chances of injury, and people who have been injured can rehabilitate their muscles much more quickly, through effective strength training.

Proper Attire

A loose-fitting shirt reduces the amount of sweat left on the bench and also the amount of body oil that touches the upholstery on the benches. Body oil causes the upholstery to become brittle and to crack. In addition, it can make the body slip on the bench. It is recommended that one carry a small towel to dry each bench after exercising on it.

---

1 W. J. Kraemer, N. D. Duncan, and J. S. Volek, "Resistance training and elite athletes: Adaptations and program considerations," *Journal of Orthopedic Sports and Physical Therapy*, August 1998, 28(2), 110–115.

2 A. Hedrick, "Resistance training with older populations: Justifications, benefits, protocol," *Strength and Conditioning Journal*, April 1998, 20(2), 32–39.

Checklist for Workout Attire

1. Wear a T-shirt or sweatshirt.
2. Wear loose-fitting or stretchable pants.
3. Wear flat tennis-shoe-type footwear to give you stability.

A T-shirt or sweatshirt helps prevent the bar from slipping during barbell squat exercises (as it may do if a tanktop is worn) and reduces the chances of bruises and scratches to the back.

Loose-fitting or stretchable pants will not rip during squats, power cleans, or hip sled exercises. Also, tight clothing may restrict circulation.

Proper footwear, such as tennis shoes rather than bare feet or sandals, gives some protection against dropped weights and stubbed toes. It also offers more stability to exercises in which the feet are a factor.[3] Elevated or flared heels, such as often found in running shoes, should not be worn because they are not as stable.

Medical Clearance

Before beginning any exercise program, you should get a medical clearance. For men, a hernia check is advised if heavy weights are to be lifted. Blood pressure should also be checked if heavy weights are to be a part of the program.

Summary

1. A fascination with weight lifting can be traced at least as far back as ancient Greece.
2. Modern scientific strength-training techniques can be traced to Dr. De Lorme's work at the time of World War II.
3. People train with weights in order to gain strength for:
   - General fitness
   - Power lifting
   - Weight lifting
   - Bodybuilding
   - Athletics
   - Recovering usage of the joints after injury
   - Developing a body that is more personally pleasing, which can increase one's self-esteem

---

3 Andrew Fry, "Proper attire," *National Strength and Conditioning Association Journal,* Dec.–Jan. 1987, 8(6), 42.

2 How to Get What You Want from Strength Training

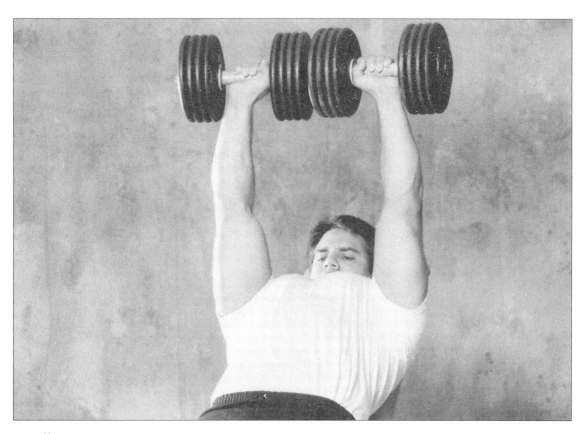

Outline

Aspects of General Fitness
Planning Your Strength-Training Program
Checklist for Terms Commonly Used
General Body Conditioning
Developing Strength
Developing Muscle Hypertrophy
Checklist for Developing Muscle Hypertrophy
Hormonal Factors
Developing Muscular Endurance
Developing Power and Speed
Plyometrics

Developing Flexibility
Developing Better Posture
Becoming a More Effective Athlete
Rehabilitating Muscles After Injury
Body Contouring
Body Measurements
Body Weight
Measuring Body Fat
Muscle Balance
Cardiovascular/Cardiorespiratory Endurance
Summary

Training with resistance—whether it be weights, springs, air- or fluid-resistance machines, or just our own body weight—not only helps us gain strength but also can change the shape of our bodies by increasing muscle size, eliminating fat, and adding definition. Some people use weights to develop power or muscular endurance for specific athletic events. Whatever your goal, the exercises are about the same. What varies are the number of repetitions, the number of sets, and the intensity and duration of the workout.

Aspects of General Fitness

The major aspects of physical fitness are strength, flexibility, and cardiovascular/cardiorespiratory (heart-blood/heart-lungs) endurance. Resistance activities are essential for gaining strength and helpful for increasing flexibility and cardiorespiratory endurance. For this reason, everyone should use resistance training as a part of a general conditioning program.

So many physical problems could be prevented if people were sufficiently strong and flexible. For example, lower back problems, one of humanity's greatest afflictions, can be reduced or eliminated in many people by proper conditioning exercises. Without sufficient strength, lifting a baby, a bag of groceries, or a piece of lumber can tear a muscle fiber and cause pain. We all need a certain degree of body conditioning and general fitness to enable us to do such everyday activities with enough reserve to protect us against injury and to make us feel good.

Planning Your Strength-Training Program

Strength develops from improved efficiency of both nerves and muscles. An efficient nervous system is able to stimulate a greater number of muscle fibers to contract at one time. It is also able to reduce the inhibition that often prevents us from exerting too much effort. It is this neural involvement that enables large gains early in a training program.

Of course, the muscles play the key role. Combined with proper nutrition and sufficient rest, strength training produces muscle fibers that are both stronger and larger and that can store more muscle fuels. The result is more efficient and harder-working muscles.[1]

But which muscles do you want to strengthen? The answer depends on why you want this strength. Do you want to be an Olympic weight lifter? Do you want to be able to throw a ball farther? To jump higher? To win at wrist wrestling? Each of these activities requires strength in several muscles. For example, if you want to be able to jump higher, you should exercise your hip extensors (your gluteal muscles), your knee extensors (quadriceps), and your

---

1 J. D. MacDougal, et al., "Biochemical adaptation of human skeletal muscle to heavy resistance training and immobilization," *Journal of Applied Physiology*, 43, 700–703.

Checklist for Terms Commonly Used

1. *Repetition* is one complete movement of a lift and return. (Example: With a barbell in both hands and at your waist, flex your elbows and bring the bar as high as it will go, then return it to the starting position.)
2. *Repetition maximum (RM)* is the number of repetitions a person can do in an exercise before the muscles are exhausted.
   - *One-repetition maximum (1 RM)* is the amount of weight that can be lifted only one time.
   - *Ten repetition maximum (10 RM)* is the amount of weight that can be lifted ten times, but not eleven.
3. *Set* is a series of repetitions—anywhere from one to more than twenty.

ankle extensors (calf muscles). You should work on each one individually and in the full coordination of a half squat, a lunge, or a leg press on a press bar, power rack, or on a weight machine. Then, of course, you should simply practice jumping.

Since an untrained person should not work with a maximum weight, you can approximate your 1 RM by finding out how much weight you can lift 10 times but not 11, then add 33 percent to that weight.

General Body Conditioning

Some strength is useful for everyone, but most of us are not looking to develop maximum strength. For general conditioning, you can do 8 to 20 repetitions with a weight. If you exercise to exhaustion, where you can't do another rep, you will get a maximum gain. If you only exercise until your muscles are rather fatigued, you will also gain something—just not as much. You determine just how fast and how far you want to go with your conditioning.

Developing Strength

If your goal is primarily to develop strength (as opposed to body contouring, for example), you will want to use a high-intensity, low-volume workout. This means that you will use a lot of weight in few repetitions or "reps" and few sets.

For your strength workout, you can do any or all of the following after a proper warm-up:

- Six to ten reps with 75 to 80 percent of your 1 RM
- Three to six reps with 85 percent of your 1 RM

- Three reps with 90 percent of your 1 RM
- One rep with maximum weight

Do one or two sets of any of the above. Or do one set of the second (three to six reps with 85 percent) and one set of the third (three reps with 90 percent).

This type of workout should teach your body to learn to contract an increasing number of muscle fibers at a time. As previously stated, the nervous system is very important to gaining strength. It is theorized that by forcing your body to lift more weight, you are probably teaching your brain to make a greater percentage of your muscle fibers contract in a short period of time. Indeed, much of the initial increase in strength experienced by beginning weight trainers is thought to be due to the training of the nerve pathways in the central nervous system.

Your muscles will probably grow larger as they get stronger, but there is no predictable correlation between muscle size and muscle strength. Some championship weight lifters show little gain in weight or size as they increase in strength.

Developing Muscle Hypertrophy

If you are working to develop muscle bulk, called *muscle hypertrophy* (hi-PER-truh-fe), your workout should be designed to make each of your individual muscle fibers larger, and your diet should be relatively high in calories, with sufficient protein and lots of carbohydrates and B vitamins. You will need to work much longer (with more sets and reps) than you would for strength, and you must plan on getting adequate rest.

Your workout will consist of low- to medium-intensity and high-volume exercise. You will work with 75 to 80 percent of your 1 RM with low to medium intensity (seven to fifteen reps) at higher volume (three to five sets). Some bodybuilders will occasionally go as high as 30 reps in a set, and may do a total of 200 reps on each muscle group in the workout period.

While you do not need the strength workout merely to develop larger muscles (which may make you look stronger), you do need it to increase your real strength. Also, an aerobic or endurance program, such as running or swimming, is necessary for maximum physical fitness, but if you include it in your workout, your bulk (hypertrophy) gains will not be as great as if you did only the bulk program.

Some women are concerned that they may develop too much muscle bulk through strength training. But because most women have less testosterone (the male hormone) than men, a greater percentage of body fat, and fewer muscle fibers, their gains in muscle hypertrophy for the same strength gains are much less than men's.[2]

While hypertrophy refers to the increase in size of the individual muscle cell, there is evidence that under extreme conditions there can be an increase in the

---

2 D. A. Lewis, E. Kamon, and J. L. Hodgson, "Physiological differences between genders: Implications for sports conditioning," *Sports Medicine*, Sept. 1986, 3(5), 357–369.

Checklist for Developing Muscle Hypertrophy

1. Select exercises that involve a large amount of muscle mass (i.e., power clean, squats).
2. Work with a 10 to 12 repetition maximum (10 to 12 RM).
3. Use high-volume training by performing multiple sets and/or multiple exercises. (Do three to four sets of each exercise and four or five different exercises for each body part you are trying to increase in size.)
4. Use short rest periods (1 to 1½ minutes).

number of cells, called *hyperplasia*. We have known for many years that this can happen in animals, and it has long been suspected to occur in humans who do very heavy strength training.

It seems that a good part of muscle hypertrophy, and probably hyperplasia, occurs during the part of an exercise where the muscle is lengthening, called the *eccentric* (ek-SEN-trik) *phase* of the exercise. Examples are returning the barbell to the resting position after a curl, or flexing the legs and hips downward at the beginning of a squat before the weight is lifted. It seems that there is more muscle fiber damage during this phase, and the damage seems to be related to increasing the size of the muscle.

We still do not have all the answers as to how muscle size occurs. Some studies suggest that bodybuilders do not seem to have larger than normal muscles,[3] whereas weight lifters and power lifters do. It has therefore been theorized that bodybuilding exercises develop more muscle fibers (hyperplasia) rather than make the individual fibers larger.

The next chapter discusses the three major types of muscle fibers. We will just say here that the three types are type I (slow-twitch) fibers, which are involved in endurance work such as running a long time; type IIb (fast-twitch) fibers, which are primarily involved in speed and power work; and, type IIa (intermediate) fibers, which are partway between the other two. Strength training can increase the size of all three, but the type of work done influences which fibers will gain the most in size. Strength training, such as that done by weight lifters and power lifters, increases the fast-twitch fiber size more. The prolonged work done by body builders increases the slow-twitch fibers and also influences the increase in the number of fibers (hyperplasia).

---

3 J. D. MacDougall, et al., "Muscle ultrastructural characteristics of elite powerlifters and bodybuilders," *European Journal of Applied Physiology*, 1982, 48, 117–126; P. A. Tesch and L. Larsons, "Muscle hypertrophy in bodybuilders," *European Journal of Physiology*, 1982, 49, 301–306.

Hormonal Factors

There are three major hormones that aid in gaining muscle bulk: testosterone (the major male sex hormone), human growth hormone (HGH), and insulin-like growth factors. Any of these present in the body will affect the ability to gain larger muscles. In addition, effective exercise increases the amount of these hormones in the body.

These muscle-growing hormones belong to a group of organic compounds called steroids. Steroids are often taken illegally by people wanting to increase their muscle size (see Chapter 12). When used, these hormones reduce the natural hormones that the exercise already produces.

Testosterone is one of the male sex hormones, or *androgens*. It aids in synthesizing protein into muscle tissue. The average man has about ten times the amount of testosterone as the average woman, but great individual variations occur naturally. Resistance training produces short-term increases in the blood testosterone level.[4] The type of exercise that seems to best promote an increase in blood testosterone levels involves large muscles (i.e., squats, power clean), heavy resistance (85 to 95 percent of 1 RM), multiple sets at medium to high volume, and short rest periods of one-half to one minute.

Human growth hormone increases protein synthesis and makes the amino acids that make up proteins more available to the cells. The body seems to produce more of this hormone with 10 RM sets for large muscles and one-minute rest periods between the sets.

Insulin-like growth factors have not been studied as extensively as the other two hormones. It seems that most exercise programs will produce an increase in these hormones in men. For women, the results are not yet conclusive.

Developing Muscular Endurance

Some athletic events, such as swimming, running, cycling, rowing, basketball, and dancing, stress cardiorespiratory endurance. Often, however, a certain muscle group tires during these activities, so it needs special work in preparation for the event. For example, a swimmer often needs extra muscular work in the shoulder area to be able to maintain speed over a longer distance. The same can be true for a cross-country runner running uphill, or a cyclist in a sprint.

Muscular endurance is achieved when more blood supply develops for the muscle and more of the muscle fibers develop extra fuel supplies, making more oxygen available to the muscle.

The workout for muscular endurance is of low intensity and high volume. Depending on the type of muscular endurance you desire, you can do 3 or 4 sets working with 40 to 50 percent of your 1 RM for 15 to 30 reps. Or you can use 25 to 30 percent of your 1 RM for 100 to 200 continuous reps.

---

4 W. J. Kraemer, "Neoendocrine response to resistance exercise," in *Essentials of Strength Training and Conditioning*, T. R. Baechle, ed. (Champaign, IL: Human Kinetics, 1994), 90–102.

Developing Power and Speed

Power is a combination of speed and strength involving the *fast-twitch* muscles (explained in Chapter 3). To develop power, you first need to develop a good deal of strength, then use that strength in an explosive way. Jumping as high as possible is one way to develop power in the legs. Maximum power seems to be generated by working quickly with 30 to 50 percent of one's 1 RM. Working against an isokinetic machine is another good way to develop power.

Speed can be similarly developed. First do exercises for strength in the muscle in which you want to develop speed. Then do the speed activity. If you want running speed, run fast in your workout. If you want swimming speed, swim as fast as possible. This is called *specificity of training*.

With the principle of "specificity of training" in mind, it should be expected that doing an exercise fast will develop more speed and power. In fact, proper speed exercise can increase the power potential of a muscle or muscle group by 300 percent.[5]

Plyometrics

Plyometric exercises are used by high-level athletes to help develop speed and power. Jumping from a 1- to 3-foot stool to the ground and immediately springing back up to another stool, or jumping rope, are examples of plyometrics for leg power. Catching and quickly throwing a medicine ball is an example of plyometrics for the arms and shoulders.

The idea of plyometrics is to make the muscle fibers contract while they are lengthening (as they do, for example, when you catch the weight). This is an eccentric contraction. More weight can be handled in an eccentric contraction. Then, while this great number of fibers is contracting, the exerciser changes the contraction to a *concentric* contraction (shortening the muscle fibers) by throwing the weight. The fibers that are already contracting eccentrically are therefore available for the concentric contraction. If the concentric contraction were performed first, not as many fibers would be called into play.

Consider another example. Jumping from a box should force a large number of muscle fibers in the thighs and calves to contract when catching the body's weight. Then, when you immediately jump upward, more muscle fibers should be available to contract concentrically, so you should be able to jump higher. Since one of the factors involved in speed, strength, or power activities is the number of muscle fibers contracting, the idea of plyometrics is to condition the muscle groups to make more fibers contract at one time.

Plyometrics should be practiced only under the direction of an expert who knows how to avoid injury to the muscles. It is an advanced training technique.

---

5 D. Hamar, "Force production characteristics of strength and power training," paper presented at the World Congress of Sports Medicine, Orlando, FL, June 2, 1998.

Guidelines for Various Strength-Training Objectives*

	Muscle Size (hypertrophy)	Strength	Power	Peak Power
Sets	3–4	3–5	3–5	1–3
Reps	8–20	2–6	2–3	1–3
Volume (total work)	High	Medium high	Low	Very low
Intensity (heavy weight)	Low	High	High	Very high

---

*Suggested by Steven Fleck, "Periodization of strength and power training," paper presented at the World Congress of Sports Medicine, Orlando, FL, June 2, 1998.

Developing Flexibility

At one time, a number of weight lifters were thought to become "muscle-bound," meaning they lacked a full range of motion for their joints. It has since been discovered, though, that the term was a misnomer, because the culprit was the tissue that holds the muscles together, not the muscles themselves. This *connective tissue* includes ligaments (which hold one bone to another), tendons (which hold a muscle to a bone), as well as the tissue that surrounds each muscle.

Connective tissue tends to lose its elasticity and to shorten as we become older.[6] However, we can manufacture more connective tissue as our muscles become stronger or larger. For that reason, it is essential that strength-training exercises involve a full range of motion—something the old so-called muscle-bound weight lifters failed to do. Today's emphasis on exercising through a full range of motion makes most strength-training enthusiasts more flexible than the average person. Ways to keep our connective tissue stretched are discussed in more detail in Chapter 6.

Developing Better Posture

Good posture results when the bones are in proper alignment and the muscles are sufficiently strong to hold them in that alignment. Generally speaking, this requires flexibility in the front of our bodies and strength in our backs and abdominals.

---

6 G. Dintiman, et al., *Discovering Lifetime Fitness* (St. Paul, MN: West, 1984), p. 255.

A forward head is corrected by stretching the front of the neck and strengthening the back of the neck.

Assuming that there is no structural abnormality, round shoulders are corrected by stretching the chest muscles that pull the shoulders forward, and by strengthening the muscles in the upper back that pull the shoulders back.

The chest is lifted by strengthening the small muscles in the lower back, which pull down on the rib cage and thus "lift" the chest.

When a "pot belly" is the result of tight connective tissue in the lower hip, it is corrected by stretching the connective tissue in the front of the lower hips and strengthening the gluteal muscles. To the degree that it is caused by an excess of fat in the diet, losing weight will be required. Usually, both factors are involved.

Specific exercises for better posture are discussed in Chapter 9.

Becoming a More Effective Athlete

Every athlete desires increased effectiveness in some area, whether it be strength, power, or the ability to develop more speed. Strength training can greatly aid in achieving these goals, but the athlete must choose the correct exercises to meet his or her goals. Which muscle groups need strength? Which joints need flexibility? Which actions need power? Which need speed? Which muscles need endurance? Exercises for each goal should be designed using the muscle in the exact range of motion and at the exact angle it is used in the athletic event.

Rehabilitating Muscles After Injury

If you have injured your muscles or joints in an accident or sports, you can bring them back to normal by using the same exercises recommended for increasing strength, flexibility, and power; but you should be under doctor's orders or following the prescription of a physical therapist.

Body Contouring

To contour your body to more desirable measurements, you will want to increase muscle bulk in some areas and to eliminate body fat. When you eliminate the fat that is just under the skin, you give your muscles more *definition*.

Of course, people are built differently. The more heavily muscled are termed *mesomorphs*, the thinner *ectomorphs*, and the fatter *endomorphs*. These basic body builds, which we inherit, are very instrumental in indicating the type of athletes we will be and how well we will respond to strength training. While few people fit any one category totally, those who are primarily mesomorphic will be able to gain more muscle bulk than those who are primarily ectomorphic. So we are not born equal in terms of our body-contouring potential.

Three body types

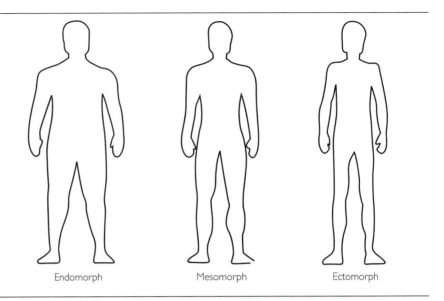

Endomorph   Mesomorph   Ectomorph

Body Measurements

To discover how you are progressing in developing muscle hypertrophy, you must get accurate measurements of several parts of your body. To do this, you must use certain standard procedures.

Body Weight

Body weight is measured on a scale. A balance scale is far more accurate than a spring-operated bathroom scale, which may be off by several pounds.

Measuring Body Fat

Just as important as body weight is the percent of body fat you are carrying. In fact, persistent dieters often increase their body fat even though their body weight does not change. Men, on the average, have between 12 and 17 percent body fat; women, between 19 and 24 percent. For men, borderline obesity is between 20 and 25 percent, and for women it is between 25 and 30 percent.[7] Body fat in male athletes is usually between 5 and 9 percent, and in female athletes between 7 and 15 percent.

Underwater (hydrostatic) weighing equipment is the most accurate (within 1 percent) for measuring body fat, but it is not often readily available.

7 J. Wilmore, *Sensible Fitness* (Champaign, IL: Leisure Press, 1986).

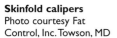
Skinfold calipers
Photo courtesy Fat
Control, Inc. Towson, MD

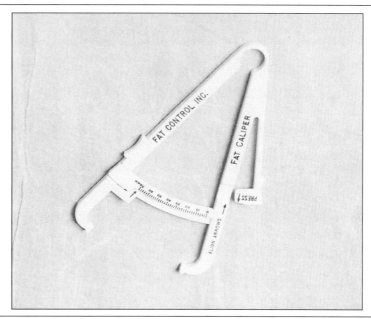

Bioelectrical impedance systems are more commonly used, although they have a greater margin of error.

Skinfold calipers, another method of measurement, are fairly accurate in the hands of an expert. Even so, the average measurement has a margin of error of 2 to 3 percent. A reading of 16 percent could actually be between 13 and 19 percent. Skinfold measurements are taken at the back of the triceps, the side front of the hips, and the front of the abdominals. (A simple caliper with complete charts can be purchased from Fat Control, Box 101 17, Towson, MD 21204.)

Girth Measurements

Girth measurements are used to mark progress in developing muscle bulk. Several body parts can be measured. Steel or cloth tapes with markings in centimeters or tenths of inches are the best measuring tools. They can be purchased at medical supply houses. Other types of flexible tapes can also be used.

The *neck* is measured with the muscles tense and the tape around the area of the Adam's apple.

The *chest* is measured after you have taken a full breath and tensed your muscles. The tape is placed just above the nipples and is parallel to the floor.

The *biceps* are measured with the elbow flexed as far as possible and the muscles tensed. Measure the largest part of the muscle belly.

The *triceps* are measured as the biceps, with the muscles tense.

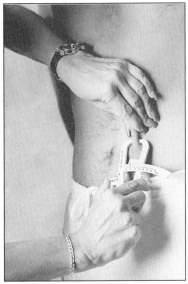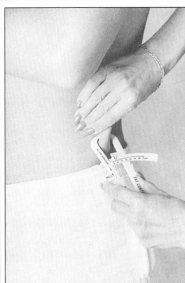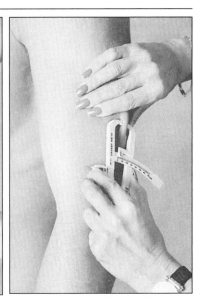

Measuring the abdomen, side, and triceps
Photos courtesy Fat Control, Inc. Towson, MD

Interpretation of the abdominal skinfold
Reproduced from Jack D. Osman, *Fat, Fat, Fat: A Threefold Look at Fat Control,* 1984

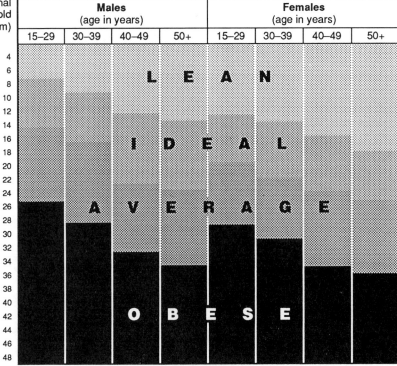

Abdominal Skinfold (in mm)	Males (age in years)				Females (age in years)			
	15–29	30–39	40–49	50+	15–29	30–39	40–49	50+
4								
6								
8			L E A N					
10								
12								
14								
16			I D E A L					
18								
20								
22								
24								
26			A V E R A G E					
28								
30								
32								
34								
36								
38								
40			O B E S E					
42								
44								
46								
48								

The *forearm* is measured at the largest part of the muscle with the muscles tensed and the fist clenched.

The *abdomen* is measured at the level of the navel after exhaling completely.

The *hips* are measured with the heels together and the buttocks tightened.

The side of the *hip* is measured just above the hip.

The *thighs* are measured while the feet are placed about 1½ feet apart. Measure the largest part of the tensed muscle—usually about 6 inches below the hip joint.

The *calves* are measured at the largest part of the muscle with the legs apart.

Muscle Balance

In exercising it is important to develop muscle balance, which means similar, but not necessarily equal, strength in the muscles that work the opposite sides of a joint. This is called *antagonistic* muscular development. It is important because if the muscles are not approximately of equal strength, the weaker muscle can be injured. So if you work the biceps, you should also work the triceps. If you work the chest, you should also work the upper back. If you work the quads, you should also work the hamstrings.

Cardiovascular/Cardiorespiratory Endurance

Cardiovascular (heart-blood) or *cardiorespiratory* (heart-lungs) endurance refers to efficient operation of the heart, circulation, and lungs. This is often called *aerobic fitness*. As you become more aerobically fit, your heart may become larger, with greater musculature and a larger blood-pumping chamber; your blood will contain more red cells and hemoglobin for carrying oxygen; and the number of blood vessels in the muscles you use in the activity (e.g., legs in runners and shoulders and arms in swimmers) may increase.

With the exception of some types of circuit training, strength workouts are not conducive to developing cardiorespiratory endurance. You should therefore develop a separate workout of running, swimming, or cycling to supplement your strength training. A good cardiovascular/cardiorespiratory workout is likely to help you to extend your lifespan by 1) reducing blood fats (triglycerides), 2) increasing your good cholesterols (heavy-density lipids), and 3) using up calories, thereby limiting the accumulation of extra body fat.

Summary

1. Strength training can be used to fulfill a number of objectives: gaining strength, bulk, power, speed, and flexibility; increasing the ratio of lean to fat tissue; becoming a better athlete; or rehabilitating injured muscles.
2. The key for each objective is to choose the proper exercises—then do them using the proper weight, with the correct technique, performed at the right

intensity, and up to the appropriate volume.

3. Choosing the proper exercise requires a decision on whether to use a dumbbell, barbell, a weight machine, an isokinetic machine, or the manual resistance of a partner or yourself. These choices are discussed in Chapters 7 and 8.

4. A 1 RM (one repetition maximum) is the amount of weight a lifter can raise one time and only one time.

5. A 10 RM (ten repetition maximum) is the amount of weight a lifter can raise ten times, but not eleven.

3 The Physiology and Biomechanics of Strength Training

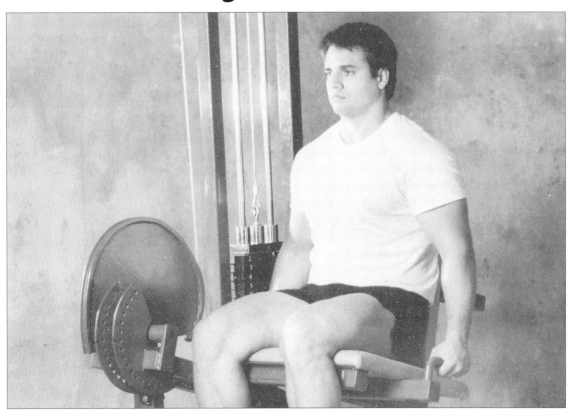

Outline

Muscles
Checklist for Understanding Muscle Fiber
Lever Action
Types of Muscular Contractions
Types of Exercises
Types of Resistance
Checklist for Buying Home Exercise Equipment
Body Positions
Joint Actions
Isolating a Muscle

Doing a Coordinated Movement
Proper Breathing
Checklist for Breathing During a Normal Strength Workout
Checklist for Breathing in Weight-Lifting Competition
Warm-Up
Checklist for Warm-Up
Soreness
Summary

Muscles

We have 434 muscle groups in our bodies that move parts of our anatomies. Only about 150 are primary movers. Each muscle is made up of thousands of individual muscle fibers having a very small diameter, from 1/300 to 1/2500 inch—much smaller than the diameter of a straight pin. (The tibialis anterior muscle in the front of the shin is estimated to have 160,000 muscle fibers.) These muscle fibers have the ability to shorten, or contract, by sliding one part of the fiber (called an *actin filament*) past another filament (called *myosin*). Each fiber either contracts totally or not at all. This is called the "all or none" principle.

There are three types of muscle fibers that can contract to move our bones:

1. Type I (sometimes called the red fibers) are slow-twitch fibers that have more blood supply and more enzymes than the other fiber types. These help in utilizing oxygen. They contract more slowly, but they also have more endurance, so they can contract many more times than the other fibers without tiring.

2. Type IIa (also called the intermediate type or the fast-twitch oxidative) is a relatively fast-twitch fiber that can pick up oxygen better than the type IIb but not as fast as the type I. In one study they were found to have five times the power of the type I fibers.[1]

3. Type IIb (white, or fast-twitch) fibers are the largest, the strongest, and act the quickest. These are the fibers most involved in strength and speed activities. In the study referenced above, these were found to have 5 times the power of the type IIa fibers, and 25 times the power of the type I fibers.

As one might expect, speed and power athletes have more fast-twitch fibers than do endurance athletes. The approximate average percentages of fast-twitch fibers for several sports follow:[2]

Sports Category	Male	Female
Marathoners	17%	
Distance runners	31%	39%
Swimmers		26%
Cross-country skiers	36%	40.5%
Cyclists	41%	49%
Bodybuilders	44%	
Downhill skiers	52%	
Untrained subjects	54%	49%
Weight lifters	60%	
Shot putters	62%	49%
Sprinters	63%	72.5%
Jumpers	63%	51.5%

1 J. J. Widrick, et al., "Force-velocity and force-power properties of single muscle fibers from elite master runners and sedentary men," *American Journal of Physiology*, August 1996, 271(2), 676–683.

2 M. Stone and H. O'Bryant, *Weight Training: A Scientific Approach* (Edina, MN: Burgess International Group, 1987), page 15.

Checklist for Understanding Muscle Fiber

1. Type I or *slow-twitch* (red) muscle fibers are used primarily for endurance. Since they use fatty acids activated by oxygen as their primary fuel, their fuel stores can be replenished by the oxygen breathed during the activity.
2. Type IIa or *intermediate* fibers use both oxygen and glycogen (a carbohydrate stored in muscle) for fuel. They are not as fast as the type IIb fibers, but they have more endurance.
3. Type IIb or *fast-twitch* (white) muscle fibers are used primarily in speed and strength contractions. They use glycogen for a fuel. They do not have many fuel stores, so they tire easily.

The number of each type of fiber is probably primarily set at birth.[3] While it appears that one type of fiber cannot be changed into another type, it is possible to condition the fibers somewhat. Specifically, endurance activity increases the ability of the type I and IIa fibers to utilize more oxygen and to contract more frequently over a period of time. In addition, some studies indicate that with enough endurance training, type IIa fibers may become more like type I fibers.

Lever Action

It is more than your muscles' force that determines how strong you can be. The way in which your bones act as levers is at least as important. Assume that two

Characteristics of the Different Types of Muscle Fibers*

Characteristic	Type I (Slow Oxidative)	Type IIa (Fast Oxidative)	Type IIb (Fast Glycolytic)
Myosin ATPase activity	Low	High	High
Speed of contraction	Slow	Fast	Fast
Fatigue resistance	High	Intermediate	Low
Oxidative capacity	High	High	Low
Anaerobic enzyme content	Low	Intermediate	High
Mitochondria	Many	Many	Few
Capillaries	Many	Many	Few
Myoglobin content	High	High	Low
Color of fiber	Red	Red	White
Glycogen content	Low	Intermediate	High
Fiber diameter	Small	Intermediate	Large

*Reprinted by permission from Dr. Steven Seiler, Agder District College, Kristensand, Norway

3 T. Rowland, *Developmental Exercise Physiology* (Champaign, IL: Human Kinetics, 1996), p. 168.

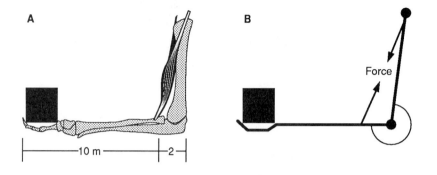

Muscle force generation and resultant torque by one of the elbow flexor muscles, the biceps humerous, over the elbow joint.

people have the same number of muscle fibers in their biceps muscles, but one has a forearm 12 inches long, with the biceps muscle attaching an inch away from the elbow joint. This is a ratio of 1 to 12. The second person has a forearm 9 inches long, with the biceps tendon attaching 1½ inches away from the elbow. This is a ratio of 1 to 6. Even though they have the same number of fibers contracting at the same time, the second person will be more than twice as strong as the first. For this reason, it is easy to see why the tall, thin basketball player will never be as strong as the short, stocky wrestler.

Types of Muscular Contractions

There are three types of muscular contractions: *concentric*, in which the muscle fiber is shortening; *static*, or *isometric*, in which the muscle is contracted but does not change its length; and *eccentric*, in which the muscle is lengthening.

In a biceps curl, as you lift the weight toward your chest, your muscles contract concentrically. If you hold the weight motionless at one point in the exer-

Biceps curl with barbell

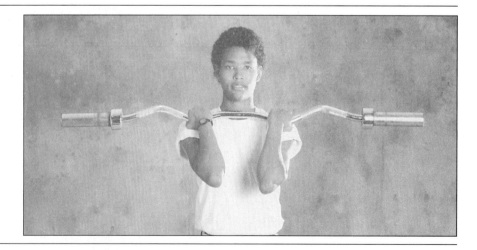

cise, your muscles will be contracting isometrically. As you let the weight return to its beginning position slowly, your muscles will be contracting eccentrically.

All three types of exercise have been advocated by different people at various times. At the present time, it is not known for certain just which type of contraction will give the lifter the greatest strength. But the consensus is that if you want strength for moving something, you probably should move something in your exercise. As mentioned earlier, greater muscle size may be gained by emphasizing the eccentric phase of the exercise.

Types of Exercises

Exercises can be classified as isotonic, isometric, or isokinetic.

Isotonic (*iso* means "same," and *tonic* means "muscle tone" or "strength") is the type of exercise done when lifting a weight such as a barbell. In an isotonic exercise, the weight stays the same during the contraction.

In *isometric* (literally means "same length") exercises, the joint does not change positions. Standing in a doorway and pushing on the jamb would be isometric. (Of course, if you break the door, the exercise would become isotonic.) This type of exercise has the lowest transfer to athletics, except for weight lifting.

Isokinetic ("same energy" or "same speed") exercises require a special type of machine that keeps the speed constant while the force is maximized. This has the highest transfer to athletic events that require speed.

If you want strength that moves things, such as on the football field or tennis court, you should do isotonic or isokinetic exercises.

Types of Resistance

The most common types of resistance are *free weights*: barbells (for two-hand exercises) and dumbbells (for one-hand exercises). These have the advantage of being relatively inexpensive and useful in many types of exercises. They also require that the lifter use other muscles than the primary lifting muscles in order to balance the weight. But they have the disadvantage of being less safe than other types of resistance systems, such as machines. If the weights are not secured properly, they may slip off. Additionally, with the heavier barbell exercises, a spotter is necessary to assist the lifter in case he or she loses balance (as in a squat) or lacks the strength to replace the weight on a rack (such as in a bench press).

Weight machines (such as Universal Gym) are safer than the free weights and also allow the resistance to be changed by simply sliding a pin to another weight. Their major disadvantage is that in some of the exercises, the lifter cannot gain as full a range of movement as can be done with free weights.

The Nautilus machines added a different element by using cams to change the resistance during the exercise. If you were using free weights to do a biceps

Chest press by Universal Gym
Photo courtesy of Universal Gym Equipment, Inc., Cedar Rapids, Iowa

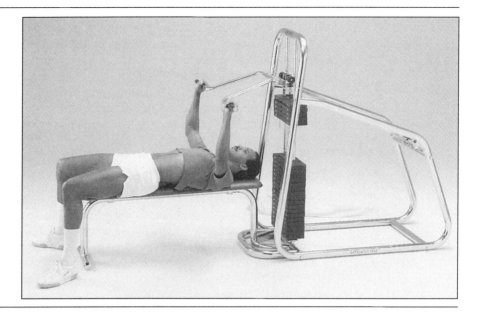

curl, it would be easy as you started the exercise but would become increasingly more difficult as you lifted the weight. By using the specially designed cam, however, you can make your muscle work harder than normal at the beginning of the exercise as well.

Resistance Weight Machines vs. Free Weights

Machines

Advantages	Disadvantages
Safer	Expensive
Many limit action to one joint	Less versatile
Easier to use	unless you have
Calibrated resistance (many	a complete set of
change resistance throughout	machines
the exercise)	Bulky, not portable
Easier to use, quicker to set	
resistance	

Free Weights (barbells and dumbbells)

Cheaper	More chance of
More variety of exercises	injury if lifts are
with each barbell or dumbbell	improperly done
	Often need a spotter
	More skill required
	(balance)

Manual resistance for triceps, arm up
(left)

Manual resistance for triceps, arm down
(right)

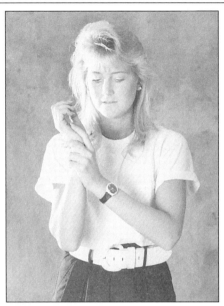 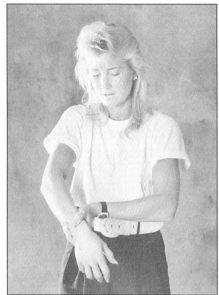

Isokinetic machines, such as Cybex or Keiser, allow the user to exert constant, or nearly constant, force against the machine. The force is measured on a gauge. This way the lifter can use full power over the entire range of motion. Also, the exercise is isokinetic, which is the best type for an athlete. Unfortunately, many people want to "pump iron" and thus overlook the benefits of working on an isokinetic machine.

Springs and *elastic bands* are often used as part of a home gym, but are seldom seen in schools or gyms. They have the advantage of being inexpensive. Their disadvantage is that their resistance increases as they are expanded, so you do not get the same level of resistance throughout the exercise.

Manual resistance from a partner or yourself (called *dynamic tension* by the famous bodybuilder Charles Atlas) is the use of one muscle against another.

 ## Checklist for Buying Home Exercise Equipment

1. Buy only from reliable wholesale or retail outlets.
2. Shop at several stores, noting the advantages and disadvantages of each piece of equipment.
3. Determine your needs and your budget.
4. Check fitness stores, Sears, or Montgomery Ward, used sports equipment shops, and the Internet for comparative prices. But buy well-made equipment. The cheapest isn't always the best deal!

There are some very real advantages in this type of resistance for some of the smaller muscles, but it is of no value in developing leg strength or bench-pressing strength. Of course, one of its greatest advantages is that it is cheap and you can't help but take your equipment with you on vacation.

Body Positions

Strength-training exercises are often described in technical anatomical terms. So lying face down is called being in the *prone* position. Lying face up is called being in the *supine* position. *Bent* means bending at the waist while standing. Other positions are *kneeling* and *standing*, which certainly need no explanation.

Joint Actions

As strength training has become more scientific, it has begun using the names for body movements that have traditionally been used in anatomy and kinesiology (the study of movement). In this book we will generally use these more scientific terms.

- *Flexion* means to decrease the angle of a joint. A biceps curl is an example of elbow flexion.
- *Extension* means to return the joint to its normal position.
- *Hyperextension* means to bring the joint to a position past normal extension.
- *Abduction* means to move a limb away from the body.
- *Adduction* means to bring the joint back from the abducted position.

Other terms are used for rotation of a joint, such as the shoulder or neck, or the complicated movements of the ankle and wrist.

Isolating a Muscle

Sometimes you will want to isolate a muscle to increase the strength of that one area. A biceps curl is an example. Sometimes you will want to isolate just one muscle group in order to remedy a weakness in a coordination. For example, suppose your bench press needs improvement. Since the bench press uses both the elbow extensors (triceps) and the shoulder-joint (arm) horizontal adductors (upper pectorals or chest), you might do a triceps extension (French curl) to strengthen that muscle, then a supine fly exercise to strengthen the upper chest and deltoids. Then you would do the bench press to check your progress in gaining the strength needed for the whole coordinated exercise.

Doing a Coordinated Movement

Most athletic movements involve several joints being moved at the same time—a multiple-joint exercise. For example, in jumping you extend the hip, knee, and ankle joints. So if you want to improve your jumping ability, you should use all three actions in one exercise. Rising from a squat position up to your toes would be one example. Or if you were using a machine such as a Universal, you would, from the sitting position, extend your leg and ankle.

Proper Breathing

There are two methods of breathing, depending on whether you are in competition or just exercising for your health.

Competitive weight lifters hold the breath against the closed glottis, called the *Valsalva maneuver*. This raises the air pressure inside the chest, thus stabilizing the upper vertebrae (thoracic section) of the backbone. As soon as the most difficult part of the lift is past, the air is exploded from the mouth as the lifter finishes the lift. The lifter then inhales when lowering the weight.

While this method generally allows for more weight to be lifted, the high air pressure in the chest increases the blood pressure significantly, sometimes to over 400 millimeters of mercury. (Normal is about 120.) If there is a weakness in the blood vessels, one may pop and hemorrhage. Another disadvantage, especially for men, is the danger of creating an inguinal hernia. When the testicles move downward from inside the body to the scrotum before birth, they weaken the tissue covering the small holes in the hips (the inguinal rings) through which they pass. The increased air pressure from lifting a heavy weight while holding one's breath can push a small part of the intestine through that opening.

The recommended method for the great majority of people is to exhale during the lifting phase of the exercise. This eliminates the potential problems of breath holding during a lift. This was first suggested in 1964[4], and is almost universally followed in strength-training classes.

---

4 R. O'Connor, "Scientific weight training," *Scholastic Coach*, Sept. 1964.

   Checklist for Breathing During a Normal Strength Workout

1. Inhale before the weight is lifted.
2. Exhale as the weight is lifted.
3. Inhale as the weight is being eccentrically lowered.

Checklist for Breathing in Weight-Lifting Competition

1. Inhale at the beginning of the lift.
2. Force the air against the glottis, not against the lips, as you start the hardest part of the lift.
3. Explode the air out of the mouth as you finish the lift.

Warm-Up

It is recommended that you warm up for your strength-training workout by doing some aerobic work such as jogging or jumping jacks. Then always begin each lift by lifting a lighter weight than planned for the exercise. However, if you plan to do an exercise for ten or more repetitions, the first few repetitions usually serve as a warm-up for that exercise. But before lifting heavy weights, do the same exercise with light weights.

Cold, unstretched muscles are much more likely to be injured than those that are warmed up. Your own age and fitness level will determine the amount of warm-up you will typically need prior to lifting.

An adequate warm-up will accomplish the following:[5]

- Increase the amount of oxygen you are taking in
- Increase the blood flow in your lungs
- Increase the rate of oxygen exchange in the muscles
- Change the blood flow from the organs and skin to the muscles
- Increase the aerobic metabolism of the muscles (the ability of the muscles to use air (oxygen) in their contractions)
- Allow for the "second wind" phenomenon to occur more rapidly in endurance activities
- Improve speed and power
- Increase the nerves' ability to transmit their impulses and to contract more muscle fibers
- Improve the range of motion of the joints
- Make you mentally ready to perform
- Possibly reduce soft tissue injuries

5 D. Wathen, "Flexibility: Its place in warm-up activities," *National Strength and Conditioning Association Journal*, Oct.-Nov. 1987, 9(5), 26–27.

Checklist for Warm-Up

1. Do a general warm-up such as jogging or jumping jacks.
2. Do specific warm-ups for each weight exercise. Five reps at 50 to 60 percent of your 1 RM will do the job.

Soreness

Soreness of the muscles generally occurs when untrained athletes work too hard. There are several possible causes. Very small injuries to either muscles or connective tissue are probably the major factor. Eccentric contractions during your exercise or such activities as running downhill or plyometrics are often the culprits. The soreness will likely last up to seven days.[6]

Summary

1. Each of our muscles is made up of thousands of tiny fibers.
2. During a muscular contraction, each of these tiny fibers either contracts totally or not at all. This is called the "all or none" principle.
3. A person can gain strength by using isotonic, isometric, or isokinetic exercise.
4. The resistance against which we work in strength-training exercises can be free weights, exercise machines, or manual resistance.
5. Exercises can be grouped according to whether they are one-joint exercises, such as a barbell curl, or multiple-joint exercises, such as a bench press.
6. The breathing style generally recommended is to exhale during the lifting part of the exercise.
7. A proper warm-up is essential.

---

6 P. Komi, P. "Neuromuscular fatigue: Disturbed function and delayed recovery after intensive dynamic exercise," paper presented at the World Congress of Sports Medicine, Orlando, FL, May 31, 1998.

4 *Choosing Your Workout Schedule*

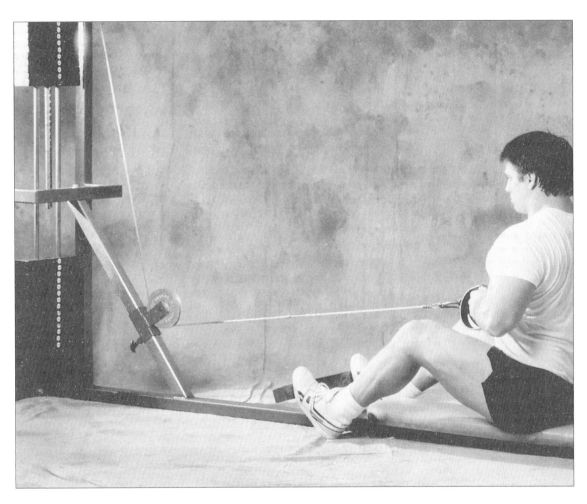

Outline

Exercise Order
Workout for Strength
Priority System
Workout for Muscle Bulk
Workout for General Body Conditioning
Rest Between Sets

Rest Between Workouts
Periodization
Recording Your Progress
Checklist for Recording Your Progress
Checklist for Workouts
Summary

There are many ways to set up a workout schedule. You can vary the exercises, such as working on squats one day, leg extensions another, and lunges on a third day. Or you can work the same sequence of exercises each day. You can work the same schedule (same weights, same number of reps and sets), or you can vary it. General guidelines for developing your schedule follow.

Exercise Order

As with your choice of exercises for your workout, your order of choosing exercises can be an individual decision. One general principle, however, is that whichever muscles you want to work on the most should be exercised early in the workout. So if you are a swimmer, you should work on the latissimus dorsi and triceps muscles first. If you are more interested in increasing your biceps strength, you should start with biceps.

If you don't have a particular muscle group in mind, the rule is to start with the complex (multiple-joint actions as shown in Chapter 8), then move to the simpler actions (the single-joint exercises shown in Chapter 7). You should also go from the larger muscles to the smaller muscles.[1]

Workout for Strength

If you are an athlete, refer to Chapter 9 for the list of strengthening exercises that are specific to your sport. (These exercises are described in detail in Chapters 7 and 8.) If you just want general strength, determine which areas of your body you want to develop. For most muscle groups, there is one "best" exercise—an exercise that gives you maximum strength and flexibility for the joint's action. The exercises for individual muscles are found in Chapter 7. If you want to be a competitive lifter or are interested in working multiple-joint actions, these exercises will be in Chapter 8.

Once you know the types of muscles and coordinated movements you want to develop, there are several choices for how you will put them together.

Priority System

In the *priority system*, you do your most important exercise first. This allows you to exhaust your muscles on that exercise before you tire yourself on the less important exercises. Be sure to work on the larger muscle groups first.

Research of many years ago indicated that three sets of five to six reps was best for strength gain.[2] Of course, your muscles should be exhausted, or at

1 W. Kraemer, "Physiological basics for resistance training programs," paper presented at the World Congress of Sports Medicine, Orlando, FL, June 2, 1998.

2 R. Berger, "Effect of varied weight training programs on strength," *Research Quarterly*, 1962, 33, 168–181.

least very tired, after each set. Well-conditioned weight trainers can generally do more work with each muscle group. Your exercise program could include this three-set, five-to-six-repetition maximum, or you can vary the reps and weight for a high-intensity workout.

Cyclic System

The *cyclic system* has proven very effective for gaining strength. The weight and number of reps will vary for each of three periods in a cycle. (The total cycle could be six to eighteen weeks, but three weeks is common.) In this type of program, the lifter does three sets of 10 RM for one part of a cycle (for three weeks of a nine-week cycle). For the next part of the cycle (another three weeks), three sets at 5 RM are done. For the last three weeks, three sets of 3 RM are done. For the next cycle, the same type of workout is repeated, but the weights are increased because the previous cycle should have increased the lifter's strength.

Pyramid System

In the *pyramid system*, the lifter starts with a lighter weight, perhaps one that can be done ten times (a 10 RM). For the next set, eight reps (8 RM), then a 6 RM, a 4 RM, a 2 RM, and finally a 1 RM. This should be followed by five or six reps with a lighter weight just to cool down.

Reverse Pyramid System

The *reverse pyramid system* starts with a warm-up, then goes immediately to a 1 RM. The lifter then reduces the weight and does a 2 RM, then 4 RM, then 6 RM, then 8 RM, and finally a 10 RM. Some experts advise against this, however, because the warm-up may not be sufficient for a true 1 RM lift so early in the workout. The gains, however, are outstanding if the muscles are exhausted at each set of RMs.

Workout for Muscle Bulk

For muscle bulk you will use less weight than for strength, but do more reps and more sets.[3] You may want to use a wide variety of exercises just to prevent boredom. But remember that there is generally one "best" exercise for each muscle group that includes isolation of the joint and maximum stretching for flexibility. (Exercise 14A on page 95 is an example of such an exercise for the triceps).

---

3 J. P. O'Shea, "Effects of selected weight training programs on the development of strength and muscle hypertrophy," *Research Quarterly*, 1966, 37, 95–102.

Two types of programs for developing muscle bulk are split routines and super sets.

Split Routines

In a *split routine*, you alternate days with different body parts. For example, on Monday and Thursday you might concentrate on legs, abdominals, and lower back, then on Tuesday and Friday you might concentrate on the upper body.

Super Sets

Super sets are often used to pump up an area of the body. For example, you might do a set of biceps curls, then follow immediately with a triceps exercise. After a short rest, you would repeat the super set, rest again, and finish with another. Super sets are generally used with the one-joint action exercises.

Workout for General Body Conditioning

Circuit training is recommended for general body conditioning. Here you go quickly from station to station with no rest. In fact, you should run in place while waiting for the next station to become available. You refrain from working at maximum because you are not seeking to be exhausted. The goal is to complete several full circuits during the exercise period. Done properly, circuit training will give your muscles a good bulk-type workout as well as condition your cardiovascular system.

For a minimal cardiovascular workout, your pulse rate should rise to approximately 150 beats per minute, the exact number varying among individuals. To find the most effective range for you, subtract your age from the number 220; this gives your maximum recommended heart rate in beats per minute. Then exercise until your heart rate is 50 to 90 percent of that number. (Various medical groups have suggested different ranges. The most commonly recommended is 60 to 90 percent of your maximum heart rate.) Work at this pace for 20 to 30 minutes.

Example: If you are 20 years old, subtract 20 from 220, which gives you 200. Take 65 percent of that 200, and you have 130 beats per minute. Take 85 percent, and you have 170 beats. So your workout should have a target heart rate range of between 130 to 170. Obviously, the 170 level would be better for your heart.

The best cardiovascular workout is continuous and rhythmic, such as running, swimming, or cross-country skiing.

The Karvonen Formula

The Finnish scientist M. J. Karvonen has improved on the simple formula of 220 minus your age as the maximum heart rate. He starts with that number, but then subtracts the resting pulse rate to determine the "heart rate reserve."

1. First take 220 minus your age ___. This is your maximum heart rate (MHR).

   Next, determine your resting heart rate while lying in bed in the morning before you get up. Use your index and middle fingers and locate your pulse, either on the side of your neck (carotid artery) or on the wrist just above the thumb. Count the number of pulse beats in a minute or take your pulse for 15 seconds and multiply by 4 to determine the total for a minute.

2. Resting heart rate (pulse rate) (rest HR) ___

3. Subtract your resting heart rate from the maximum pulse rate.

   MHR ___ – rest HR ___ = ___ heart rate reserve (HRR)

   Now you will determine your maximum and minimum pulse rates for an effective workout. For the average person, your high end will be your heart rate reserve multiplied by 80 percent (.80) added to your resting pulse rate.

4. ___(HRR) × .80 = ___ + ___ (rest HR) = ___ maximum desirable heart rate during exercise

   Next find the minimal acceptable level for your workout by multiplying your heart rate reserve (HRR) by 60 percent (.60), added to your resting pulse rate.

5. ___ (HRR) × .60 = ___ + ___ (rest HR) = ___ minimal desirable heart rate during exercise

   These two percentages (60 and 80 percent) are not set in stone. If you have medical problems or are in very poor condition, you might use a number between 40 and 55 percent to set your minimal pulse rate. If you are very fit or a competitive athlete, you might use 85 or 90 percent to set your high-end exercise pulse rate.

   Here is an example of how a 20-year-old would determine her target training pulse range. Assume that her resting pulse rate is 70.

   Minimum target heart rate (220 – 20 = 200 – 70 = 130) × .60 = 78 + 70 = 148

   Maximum target heart rate (220 – 20 = 200 – 70 = 130) × .80 = 104 + 70 = 174

   For a 40-year-old with a resting pulse of 65, the target heart rates would be:

   Minimum target heart rate (220 – 40 = 180 – 65 = 115) × .60 = 69 + 65 = 134

   Maximum target heart rate (220 – 40 = 180 – 65 = 115) × .80 = 92 + 65 = 157

Rest Between Sets

You must rest, but not too long, between sets. Generally, if you are doing an isolated movement such as a biceps curl or a triceps exercise, 1 to 1½ minutes is sufficient time for a rest. For a multi-joint exercise such as a press or a squat, 2 to 3 minutes (maximum) should be enough.

The fewer reps you are doing to exhaustion, the longer the recommended rest period is. So a 2 RM set will require a longer rest than a 6 RM set. However, if you are working with lighter weights to develop endurance, your rest periods should be much shorter.

Rest Between Workouts

Rest is essential for developing muscles. This is the reason that strength-training programs are generally done only every other day, while endurance exercises such as swimming or running can be done daily. Highly trained weight lifters, however, can lift daily if they replace the glycogen adequately during a 24-hour rest period.

The rest period does two things. It allows the body to repair the small damages to the muscle fibers, and allows the lactate and hydrogen ions (by-products of the exercise) to stimulate the pituitary gland to secrete more human growth hormone.[4] This strongest of the natural steroids helps to increase muscle size.

Periodization

Periodization is important for those wishing to make maximum gains in strength or hypertrophy. It refers to changing the type or the intensity of the exercise for different periods of the year as follows:[5]

- Microcycle—a one- to four-week period of training
- Mesocycle—a period of three or four microcycles
- Macrocycle—the largest division of a training year, including three periods: preparation (strength-gaining and hypertrophy phase), competition (strength maintenance with high intensity and low volume), and transition (recovery and maintenance phase). The macrocycle can be as short as six months but usually lasts a year—from the major competition (such as the national championships) to the next major competition (the next year's national championships). Some athletes might use a four-year cycle geared to Olympic competition.

---

4 W. Kraemer, "Physiological basics for resistance training programs," paper presented at the World Conference on Sports Medicine, Orlando, FL, June 2, 1998.

5 National Strength and Conditioning Association Roundtable, "Periodization," *National Strength and Conditioning Association Journal*, Oct.–Nov. 1986, 8(5), 12–22.

Periodization allows for different types of peak performances. It also allows for changes in workouts to reduce boredom (which might reduce an athlete's drive to excel). It requires changes in intensity and volume. *Intensity* refers to how close you are working to the maximum amount of weight you can handle (close to 1 RM). *Volume* refers to the amount of work done (the total amount of weight lifted in a workout).

Rest and restoration periods are also important parts of each period. Performance will be improved if the rest periods are adequate to allow the body and mind to recover from the fatigue of the workout schedule.

Recording Your Progress

When setting up your workout, you will need to determine which exercises you will do, how much weight you will use, how many repetitions you will perform, and how many sets of each exercise you will do. Then you will be prepared to make out your strength-training record card as follows:

Name Date	Reps/Weight	Reps/Weight	Reps/Weight	Reps/Weight	Reps/Weight	Reps/Weight
Squats						
Bench Press						
Lats						
Curl-ups						
Back Extension						
Quads						
Hamstrings						
Hip Adductors						
Biceps						

1. On the left side of the card, list the exercises you will perform.
2. Early in your program, you will have to experiment with the weight until you can estimate your 1 RM or 10 RM.
3. Determine what weight you will work with for each exercise. For most people in a general conditioning program, a set of 8 to 12 reps is adequate. So select a weight and lift it as many times as you can. If you cannot do 8 reps, the weight is too heavy. If you can do more than 12, it is too light.
4. Perform the exercise, then record the weight used and the number of repetitions. Record each set separately. For example, for a strength workout, your card might look like this for one day:

Name	Date					
	Reps/Weight	Reps/Weight	Reps/Weight	Reps/Weight	Reps/Weight	Reps/Weight
Squats	7/190	8/190	8/190	10/190	7/200	7/200
Bench Press	10/150	8/160	9/160	9/160	10/160	7/170
Lats	9/50	9/50	10/50	7/55	8/55	8/55
Curl-ups	10/0	8/5	9/5	10/5	8/10	9/10
Back Extension	6/0	8/0	12/0	6/5	7/5	7/5
Quads	9/50	9/50	10/50	7/60	8/60	8 160
Hamstrings	8/40	8/40	8/40	9/40	9/40	9/40
Hip Adductors	10/20	8/25	8/25	9/25	10/25	7/30
Biceps	7/90	8/90	9/90	9/90	10/90	7/100

If you are working for hypertrophy, the number of reps will probably be the same for every set, because you are not trying to exhaust your muscle through maximum work as in the strength exercises. So your record might look like this: 165/15, 165/15, 165/15. Or if the number of sets is always the same, perhaps three or five sets, you might just mark your typical set 165/15, and you will know that you performed three or five sets with that weight. It can also be written as sets × reps × weight, as follows: 3 × 15 × 165.

 Checklist for Recording Your Progress

1. List the exercises that you will perform.
2. Find your 1 RM (repetition maximum).
3. Determine how much weight you will lift.
4. Record the weight lifted, the number of repetitions, and the number of sets completed.

Checklist for Workouts

Priority Workout

For the priority workout, select the muscle groups that you are most interested in developing, and work on them first.

- Priority of legs, chest, biceps, triceps
- Priority of chest, biceps, triceps, legs

Cyclic Progression

Rather than using a standard workout of three sets of six to eight repetitions each time over a ten-week period, you might divide that ten weeks into cycles of three or four weeks and change the amount of weight and the number of repetitions for each cycle.

- Weeks 1 through 3: three sets of ten reps (using a 10 RM)
- Weeks 4 through 7: three sets of five reps (using a 5 RM)
- Weeks 8 through 10: three sets of three reps (using a 3 RM)

Pyramid Workout

After warming up with about 50 percent of the 1 RM, start with more repetitions of a lighter weight and work towards the 1 RM. An example with approximate weights and repetitions follows:

- 70 percent of 1 RM for ten reps
- 80 percent of 1 RM for five reps
- 90 percent of 1 RM for three reps
- 95 percent of 1 RM for two reps
- Maximum weight one rep

Reverse Pyramid

After warming up, start with a 1 RM, reduce the weight, and increase the reps for each succeeding set. An example follows:

- 1 RM
- 90 percent of 1 RM for three to five reps
- 80 percent of 1 RM to exhaustion
- 70 percent of 1 RM to exhaustion

Weight can continue to be reduced for more sets.

Split Routines

The lifter works the upper body one day and the lower body the next. (Abdominals should be worked every day.) Split routines can be done four, five, or six days a week, depending on the physical condition of the lifter and the strength of his or her motivation. Examples follow:

	Day 1	Day 2	Day 3	Day 4	Day 5	Day 6	Day 7
4 workouts per week	lower	upper	rest	lower	upper	rest	rest
5 workouts per week	lower	upper	lower	upper	lower	rest	rest
(next week)	upper	lower	upper	lower	upper	rest	rest
6 workouts per week	upper	lower	upper	lower	upper	lower	rest

(continued)

Super Sets

Super sets exercise one muscle group, then the antagonistic group.
Examples follow:

- Biceps curls/triceps extensions
- Bench press/bent rows
- Standing (military) press/lat pull-downs
- Leg extension (quadriceps)/leg curl (hamstrings)
- Abdominal curls/back extensions
- Hip abduction/hip adduction

Periodization

The length of each microperiod within a macroperiod can vary. Here is an
example of a 12-week macroperiod:

Period	Objective	Workout	Period Length	Sets/ Reps
1	Hypertrophy	High volume (high reps) Low intensity (low weight)	4 weeks	3/10
2	Strength	Moderate volume (moderate reps) Medium intensity (medium weight)	4 weeks	3/5 Target weight 1/10 70% of target weight
3	Power	Low volume (low reps) High intensity (high weight)	4 weeks	2/3 Medium weight 3/3 Target weight 1/10 70% of target weight
4	Rejuvenation	Very low volume (few reps)	2 weeks	No organized strength work; play games, do aerobic activities

Summary

1. Your strength-training program must be designed to meet your individual goals.
2. Select exercises to meet those goals.
3. Estimate your 1 RM (repetition maximum) for each exercise. Do not attempt a 1 RM until you have worked out at least three weeks.
4. Determine the intensity level you wish to use in your workout and adjust your RM to that intensity. For example, for every repetition in excess of 1, reduce the weight lifted by 2.5 percent.
5. Determine the proper routine for exercises and for rest time between exercises and between each workout.
6. For strength you will probably choose a priority, pyramid, or a cyclic program.
7. For hypertrophy you might choose to do super sets or a split routine.
8. Periodization is a workout system for serious weight trainers that changes the type of workout throughout the period and allows the athlete to peak at a certain time during the cycle.

5

The Mental Approach to Strength Training

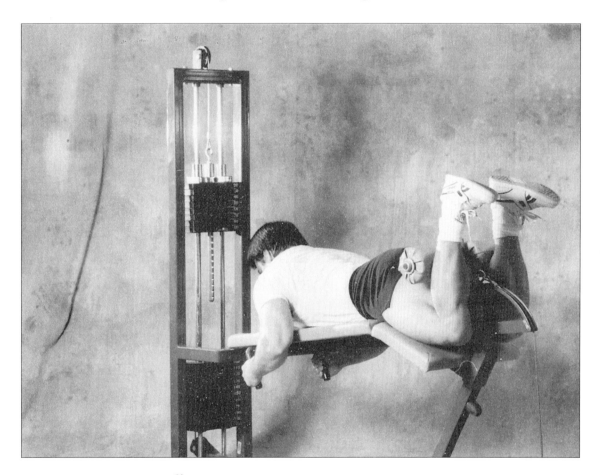

Outline

Setting Goals

The Mental Benefits of Strength
  Training

Imagery

Checklist for Mental Imagery

Relaxation

Concentration

Mental Training Works

Rehearse Success

Summary

There is an important side of strength training which is mental rather than physical. The mental aspects of strength training include:

1. *Setting goals* and developing the proper intensity of motivation.
2. Taking advantage of the *mental benefits* that result from the release of endorphins (which produce a feeling of pleasure).
3. Using *mental imagery* to increase the ability to lift weights.
4. Learning to *concentrate* at certain times during the workout and at specific times during competition.
5. Learning to *relax* between exercises and during competition.

Setting Goals

Typical goals for a strength-training program are:

- To develop general strength fitness for everyday living
- To develop strength in an injured joint
- To contour the body so that it looks more attractive
- To increase lean body mass and reduce body fat
- To develop better posture
- To develop strength and techniques specifically for weight-lifting competitions
- To develop muscular endurance
- To develop more speed and power
- To develop strength specifically for improved athletic performance

The intensity and extent of one's desire to accomplish any of these goals is called *motivation*. The degree of motivation can be measured by how fervently the goal or goals are pursued. It has been said that "a person isn't what he says, but rather what he does."

The Mental Benefits of Strength Training

A higher level of physical fitness helps people feel better and cope better with mental stresses.[1] Their self-concept is enhanced not only by the development of a better physique, but also by the feeling of success that comes from accom-

---

1 C. H. Folkins and W. E. Sime, "Physical fitness training and mental health," *American Journal of Psychology*, 1981, 36, 373–389.

Checklist for Mental Imagery

1. See yourself from the outside as you make an imaginary lift. Is the technique correct?
2. Feel the imaginary lift from the inside. Imagine that the weight feels lighter.
3. Imagine yourself doing a 1 RM with a weight heavier than that which you have been able to lift. Concentrate on lifting it—and feel yourself doing it.

plishing goals set.[2] Both men and women who are stronger and more physically fit have better self concepts.[3]

Imagery

Imagery, or *visualization*, is mental practice. Much of the early work in developing the technique was done in the United States, but it was the Eastern block countries that refined and applied this knowledge. The basic principles, however, have been instinctively employed to some degree by many athletes for years.

In visualization, the user can see the activity from the outside or feel it from the inside. Jack Nicklaus, the famous golfer, explains the visualization process of himself as "going to the movies." He just closes his eyes and sees himself performing his swing.

Greg Louganis, the Olympic champion diver, started his mental practice of a dive with the same kind of external visualization, then he *felt* himself doing the dive—internal visualization. He also found it helpful to play appropriate music while he mentally performed the dive.

You can apply these techniques to lifting by first picturing yourself doing the exercise correctly, then feeling yourself doing it. If you are trying to increase your maximum lift, you should imagine yourself lifting a weight higher than your 1 RM.

2 L. A. Tucker, "Self-concept a function of self-perceived somatotype," *Journal of Psychology*, 1983, 113, 123–133; "Muscular strength and mental health," *Journal of Personality, Sociology, and Psychology*, 1983, 45, 1355–1360; "Effect of weight training on self-concept: A profile of those influenced most," *Research Quarterly*, 1983, 54, 389–397.

3 J. B. Holloway, "Self-efficacy and training for strength in adolescent girls," Master's thesis, University of Southern California, 1985.

Relaxation

Everyone can benefit from learning to relax more effectively. Hindu yogis have practiced the art of relaxation for thousands of years, and it continues to be regarded as a worthwhile pursuit today. Recently a Harvard University medical doctor, Herbert Benson, developed a simple technique of relaxation in which one simply sits in a chair, loosens one's clothes, closes the eyes, and breathes deeply while shutting out extraneous thoughts.[4]

Shutting out the thoughts while breathing deeply is the key element. Benson suggests repeating slowly a nonsense syllable with each breath. You might say "one, one, one" or "om, om, om" as you inhale or exhale. Although other thoughts will come into your head, if you just keep repeating the nonsense syllable, those thoughts will leave. This type of relaxation has been shown to reduce stress and lower blood pressure.

Once you have become accomplished at the technique of relaxation, you can do it standing or sitting. In fact, many runners have learned to relax during their competition.

Since stress creates tension and uses energy, it will reduce one's strength. For this reason, it is important to be able to relax effectively between sets and before competition.

Concentration

When you concentrate, you narrow the focus of your thought power to one object or task, or even just one element of an object or task. Thus, a golfer may concentrate on just one small part of the golf ball before swinging to hit it. A weight trainer may concentrate on the pressure against the hands or on one muscle group before and during the exercise. This kind of concentration is often called *focusing*.

A weight trainer should concentrate on some area of every repetition, but should concentrate more fully on the more important ones. During competition, special concentration might be needed on the last set or on a lift.

Mental Training Works

Dr. Charles Garfield relates his experience as the subject of an experiment in the mental approach to weight lifting.[5] As a weight lifter who met several Soviet psychologists at an international meeting, he doubted the validity of the results the Soviets had reported.

---

4 H. Benson, *The Relaxation Response* (New York: Morrow, 1975).

5 C. Garfield, *Peak Performance* (Los Angeles: Tarcher, 1984).

The Soviets asked him about his maximum bench press. He said it was 365 pounds, done eight years earlier when he was in serious training. They asked his most recent bench press max, and he said 280. Then they asked how long he thought it would take to train to again reach his maximum. He said, "At least nine months." With this information the Soviets were ready to prove their position.

They asked him to attempt a 300-pound press. To his great surprise, he succeeded—barely. Then they directed his relaxation using advanced techniques and had him deeply relaxed for 40 minutes. They added 65 pounds to the bar and had him visualize lifting it. They had him mentally rehearse every aspect of the lift, from the feeling in the muscles to the sounds that he made while lifting. The process was repeated until he felt totally confident in what was about to happen. He concentrated on the lift and made it—equaling his lifetime best.

Rehearse Success

In any mental rehearsal, whether for a life goal or a strength-training goal, it is essential to think positively. Concentrating on failure will produce it. If you concentrate on success, you are, in effect, practicing to succeed.

Summary

1. Strength training, like other types of physical exercise, can promote a feeling of well being.
2. Strength trainers and weight lifters must set specific goals in order to know what tasks they should perform.
3. One's motivation is the intensity of one's desire to accomplish a goal.
4. Strength trainers can benefit from the mental techniques that have been used in so many other sports.
5. Visualization of the lift can be external—"seeing" yourself performing it in your mind's eye—or internal—"feeling" yourself performing it.
6. Relaxation is necessary to reduce tension between sets during workouts and between lifts during competition.
7. Concentration can increase the amount of weight lifted in an exercise.

6 *Flexibility Exercises*

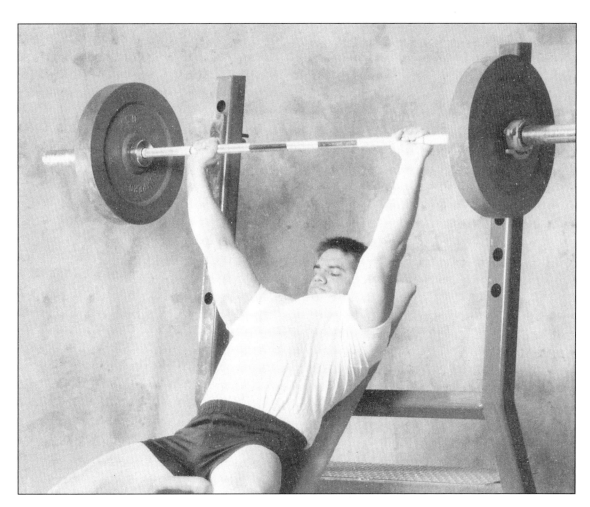

Outline

Shoulder and Chest

Groin

Lower Back and Hamstrings

Trunk

Thigh and Groin

Calf

Triceps

New Research on Stretching

Checklist for Workout Progression

Summary

Flexibility is generally defined as the range of motion of a joint It is related to the length of various connective tissues in the joints, such as the ligaments and tendons. Every weight lifter and athlete needs a certain amount of flexibility. Indeed, studies have found that Olympic gymnasts and weight lifters are the most flexible athletes.

Stretching exercises should be done very slowly. Then the stretch can be held (a *static* stretch) or the movement can continue (a *ballistic* or *dynamic* stretch), but movements should never be jerky. The PNF (proprioceptive neuromuscular facilitation) exercises have been found to be the most effective. In this type of exercise, a partner applies pressure to help the person stretching achieve a greater amount of stretch.[1]

Begin your flexibility warm-up by raising the body's temperature a bit with light cardiovascular exercise such as jogging, stationary cycling, or the Stairmaster. Follow with a few simple flexibility exercises to stretch your connective tissues and your muscles so that they will be more ready to react efficiently and less likely to be injured during the strength workout. The preferred order for stretching exercises is as follows:

- Shoulder and chest
- Groin
- Lower back and hamstrings
- Trunk
- Thigh and groin
- Calf
- Triceps

Shoulder and Chest

1. *Shoulder rotation.* Stand erect with your arms extended out to your sides. Rotate them forward in circles, your hands making circles of 12 to 15 inches. Do this for 15 seconds, then rotate them backward for 15 seconds.

2. *Seated shoulder and chest stretch.* Sit on the floor with your legs together and flat on the floor and with your body erect. "Walk" your hands backward to a comfortable stretch position. Concentrate on keeping your upper body straight and stretching the tissue in the front of your shoulder. Hold this position for 20 to 30 seconds.

---

1 Coaches' Roundtable, "Prevention of athletic injuries through strength training and conditioning," *National Strength and Conditioning Association Journal*, 5(2), 14–19; Coaches' Roundtable, "Flexibility," *NSCA Journal*, 6(4), 10–22; S. P. Sady, et al., "Flexibility training: Ballistic, static, or proprioceptive neuromuscular facilitation?" *Archives of Physical Medicine Rehabilitation*, 63, 261–263.

Groin stretch (3)

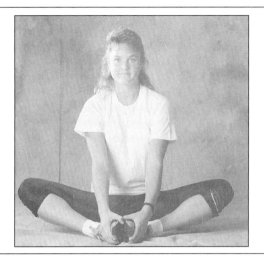

Groin

3. *Groin stretch.* While seated on the floor, put the soles of your feet together and pull them toward your hips with your hands until the heels are about 15 inches from your hips.. With your back straight, try to press your knees to the floor. Do this for 20 to 30 seconds.

Lower Back and Hamstrings

4. *Lower back and hamstrings.* While sitting on the floor, spread your legs outward as far as possible. While keeping your back and legs straight, with your toes pointed up, reach your hands as far as possible toward your right ankle. Do this for 20 to 30 seconds, then repeat with your left ankle.

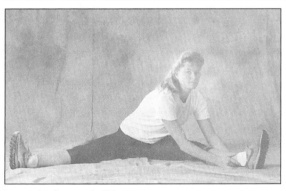 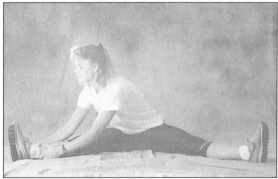

Lower back stretch (4)

Gluteal stretch (5)

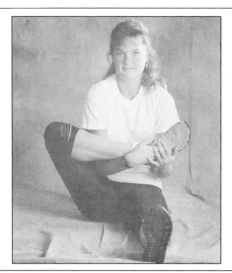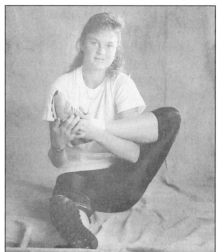

5. *Gluteal stretch.* Sit on the floor with your legs together and flat on the floor. Grab your right heel with your left hand, pass your right arm under your right calf, and lift your right foot toward the midsection of your body.

Trunk

6. *Trunk twist.* While sitting on the ground with your legs straight, bend your right leg and cross it over your left leg, and put your right foot flat on the ground. Reach your left arm around your bent leg as if you were tying to

Sitting trunk twist (6)

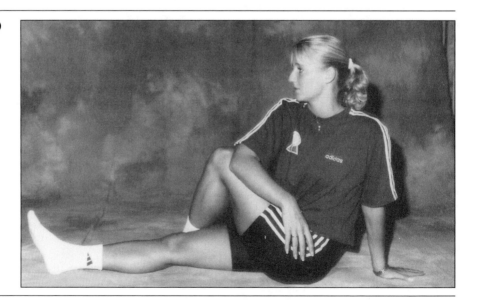

**Standing trunk twist
(7)**

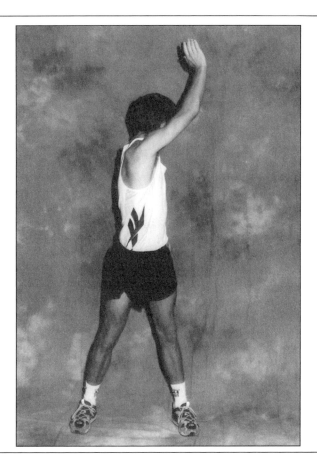

touch your hip. Place your right arm behind you as you slowly twist your head and neck until you are looking over your right shoulder. Hold for 30 seconds, then repeat for the other side.

7. *Standing trunk twist.* Reach up and twist as far as possible.

Thigh and Groin

8. *Thigh and groin stretch.* From a standing position, step forward with your left leg. Lean forward over your left leg while keeping your left foot flat on the floor. Keep your torso upright. Push down with your right leg until you feel a good stretch in your right thigh and groin area. You can put your hands on the ground for balance. Stretch for 30 seconds, then repeat with the other leg.

Thigh and groin stretch (8)

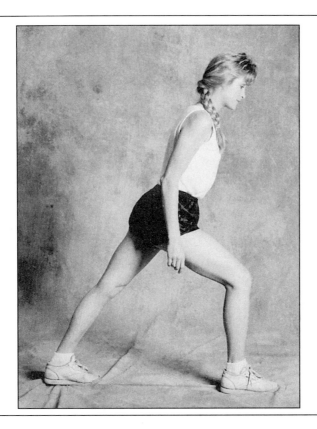

Calf

9. *Calf stretch.* From a standing position, bend your torso forward and push your right heel to the ground. You should feel the stretch in the back of the heel.

Triceps

10. *Triceps and lats stretch.* While standing, pull your right elbow behind your head until you feel the stretch. Hold for 30 seconds, then repeat with the other arm.

11. Triceps stretch. With your left hand, pull your right elbow across your chest. Hold for 30 seconds.

New Research on Stretching

While traditionally it has been common to stretch prior to physical activity, recent research indicates that stretching before the workout is not always recommended. It may increase the risk of injury and reduce one's potential strength.[2] Distance runners are currently studied more often than other athletes in terms of the desirability of stretching. So far, the results indicate that for long-distance running, stretching may not be effective as an injury preventive.

A 1983 survey of 500 runners found that those who warmed up had more injuries than those who did not (87.7 percent versus 66 percent), and the frequency of injuries increased with the length of the warm-up.[3] And a survey of 10K runners found that those who stretched had more injuries, although it is not known whether those who stretched did so because they already had an injury.[4] In a year-long study of recreational distance runners, it was found that those who occasionally stretched had more injuries than those who always stretched or those who never stretched. Those who never stretched, however, had fewer new injuries than those who stretched.[5] While the above studies cast doubt on the effectiveness of stretching for distance runners, certainly more and better research needs to be done.

In some activities, you can stretch too long or too far in your warm-up. For example, if you are entering a sprint race, on the track or in the pool, you would want your muscle fibers to be tighter and "stiffer"; too much stretch can slow you down. This is also true of jumpers—high jump or long jump—as well as swimmers and weight lifters. But if you are getting ready for a tennis match, a long run, or a leisurely afternoon of skiing, stretching is probably not harmful.[6]

More research is now being conducted into the effectiveness of warm-up stretching for various types of activities. With this newer research in mind, we can say that stretching before a strength-training workout should not be a problem. If you are in a weight-lifting competition, however, precompetition stretching might reduce your strength. Instead, stretching after your workout, when the connective tissues are warmer, should increase your flexibility effectively.

Research on stretching has not answered all, or even most, of our questions on whether to stretch or how to stretch. Is stretching a poor warm-up for a distance runner but a necessary factor for a high jumper or dancer? At present, we don't know for certain. One thing we do know is that we are all individuals with individual potentials or problems relative to our muscles and connective tissues. Some people like to do stretching exercises as part of their warm-up,

2 G. W. Gleim and M. P. McHugh, "Flexibility and its effects on sports injury and performance," *Sports Medicine* [New Zealand], Nov. 1997, 24(5), 289–299.

3 J. A. Kerner and J. C. D'Amico, "A statistical analysis of a group of runners," *Journal of the American Podiatry Association*, 1983, 73(3), 160–164.

4 S. J. Jacobs and B. L. Berson, "Injuries to runners: A study of entrants to a 10,000 meter race," *American Journal of Sports Medicine*, 1986, 14(2), 151–155.

5 S. D. Walter, et al., "The Ontario cohort study of running-related injuries," *Archives of Internal Medicine*, 1989, 149(11), 2561–2564.

6 G. Wilson, "Applied resistance training: A scientific approach," work in preparation.

✓   *Checklist for Workout Progression*

1. Do a general body warm-up such as jogging, running in place while swinging your arms, or stationary cycling.
2. If you feel more comfortable doing stretching exercises, do the stretches specified in this chapter.
3. Perform each resistance exercise with a lighter weight than you will use in the workout.
4. Perform your resistance exercise with the proper amount of weight and for the appropriate number of repetitions.
5. For a more permanent gain in flexibility, do the stretching exercises after your workout.

---

some do not. You may need to experiment with stretching versus non-stretching in your warm-up. If you stretch, you may want to experiment with the types of stretches you do and whether you stretch to the maximum degree possible.

Finally, it is known that for strength training, especially when attempting to lift the maximum weight, it is essential to lift lesser amounts of weight to warm up the muscles.

Summary

1. Stretching exercises help you achieve a full range of motion.
2. Stretches should be held at least 15 seconds and are more effective if held 30 seconds.
3. Stretches should be done slowly and held at the maximum stretching position (static stretch); or movement may be continued (dynamic or ballistic stretch), but should never be done in jerky motions.
4. Stretches are very effective when done with the aid of a partner (PNF-proprioceptive neuromuscular facilitation).
5. When stretches are done after a workout, the stretching is more likely to give a longer lasting effect of flexibility.
6. For some kinds of activities, stretching is not recommended as a warm-up.

7   *Single-Joint (Isolation) Exercises*

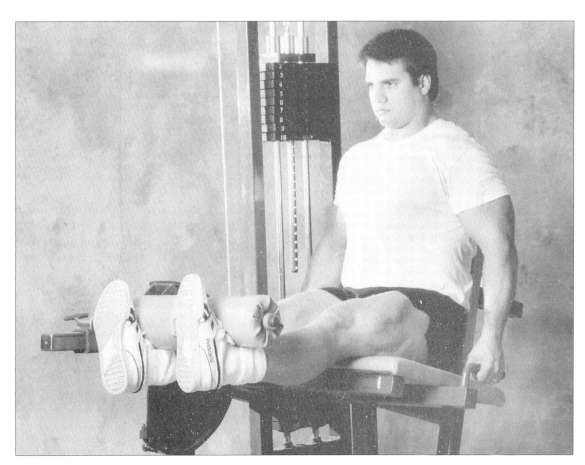

Outline

Determining the Desired Outcome
Selecting the Exercises
Selecting the Equipment
Isolating the Joint Action
Checklist for Abdominal Exercises
Summary

I n choosing the exercises for your workout, you must decide whether you want to isolate an action (as in a supine fly for the upper chest and front deltoids, or a triceps extension for the triceps) or work on a combination of actions (as in a bench press). If you want to strengthen your abdominal muscles, for example, you are concerned with only one joint action. If you want to be able to jump higher, you will be concerned with a number of muscles—the hip and knee extensors, which straighten the legs; the calf muscles, which extend your ankles; and a number of other muscles that aid in your jump.

This chapter deals with exercises that isolate one joint action. The next chapter discusses exercises which use several joint actions together—the compound exercises. For maximum strength, you will want to do both kinds of exercises. For example, if you are a basketball player who wants to be able to jump higher, you will want to work each individual muscle that you will use in jumping, then combine them in the total jumping action such as a squat or a plyometric exercise.

Determining the Desired Outcome

Are you working for strength, bulk, flexibility, or muscular endurance? Do you want to acheive better posture and body toning, or improve your performance in a specific athletic event? You will approach your program differently depending on the desired outcome. For example, if you are trying to improve your posture, you will need flexibility exercises for the front of your torso (shoulders and hips) and some strength and muscular endurance for the muscles in the back. If you want to improve in an athletic event, your workout will be characterized by more intensity (higher weight resistance) than that of a person who wants only general fitness.

Selecting the Exercises

As mentioned, this chapter presents single-joint exercises. Determine which muscles you want to develop, then select the appropriate exercise. Often you will have more than one choice.

Selecting the Equipment

Your next task is to select your equipment. You are limited, of course, by the equipment available to you. If you have only free weights, it will be more difficult for you to work effectively on the muscles below the shoulders, because you will not be able to use pulleys. Or, if you will be working out at home but have no weights, you will have to do manual resistance (or "dynamic tension") exercises in which you work one of your muscles against another.

Another thought to keep in mind is that for most people, strength gain is very specific. You will generally gain strength at the exact angle at which you

Muscles of the Body

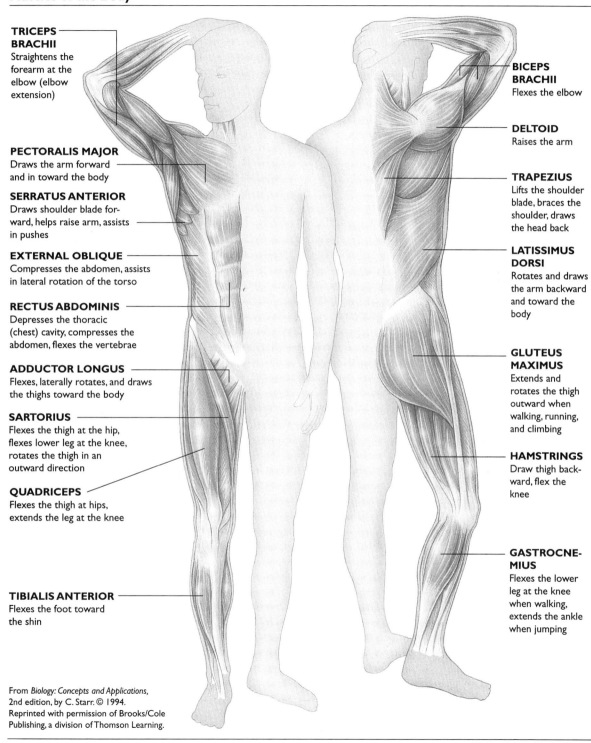

TRICEPS BRACHII
Straightens the forearm at the elbow (elbow extension)

PECTORALIS MAJOR
Draws the arm forward and in toward the body

SERRATUS ANTERIOR
Draws shoulder blade forward, helps raise arm, assists in pushes

EXTERNAL OBLIQUE
Compresses the abdomen, assists in lateral rotation of the torso

RECTUS ABDOMINIS
Depresses the thoracic (chest) cavity, compresses the abdomen, flexes the vertebrae

ADDUCTOR LONGUS
Flexes, laterally rotates, and draws the thighs toward the body

SARTORIUS
Flexes the thigh at the hip, flexes lower leg at the knee, rotates the thigh in an outward direction

QUADRICEPS
Flexes the thigh at hips, extends the leg at the knee

TIBIALIS ANTERIOR
Flexes the foot toward the shin

BICEPS BRACHII
Flexes the elbow

DELTOID
Raises the arm

TRAPEZIUS
Lifts the shoulder blade, braces the shoulder, draws the head back

LATISSIMUS DORSI
Rotates and draws the arm backward and toward the body

GLUTEUS MAXIMUS
Extends and rotates the thigh outward when walking, running, and climbing

HAMSTRINGS
Draw thigh backward, flex the knee

GASTROCNE-MIUS
Flexes the lower leg at the knee when walking, extends the ankle when jumping

From *Biology: Concepts and Applications*, 2nd edition, by C. Starr. © 1994. Reprinted with permission of Brooks/Cole Publishing, a division of Thomson Learning.

work. For example, suppose you are a football lineman, and you work on the bench press at a 90-degree angle to your body. In a game, however, you use your arms at a 110-degree angle. Since your maximum strength is at the 90-degree angle, you will not benefit fully from that exercise. To solve this problem, you need to exercise the muscle at all the angles where you want your maximum strength. An incline press would be more effective.

As another example, in a biceps curl your muscles work at different intensities from the beginning of the exercise through the finish. The amount of force required changes with each degree of flexion of your elbow. This can be corrected by exercising on an isokinetic machine (such as Cybex), a hydrolic or air machine (such as Hydrafitness or Keiser), or a machine using cams (such as Nautilus). The problem with isokinetic machines is that the lifter has to push as hard as possible to get maximum gains, so it is easier to "cheat" by not working to the maximum.

Next, decide whether you are going to work for strength (1 to 7 reps with 80 to 100 percent of your 1 RM), bulk (7 to 15 reps with 75 to 80 percent of your 1 RM), or muscular endurance, in which you might do 20 to 100 reps with a weight.

For most athletic events, you will want to develop strength, speed, and power. If looking good at the beach is your objective, you will probably opt for muscle bulk. Most people who want muscular endurance are better off doing a general body aerobics activity such as running, swimming, or cycling rather than lifting weights. However, weights can have their place in a muscular-endurance program. For example, if you are a skier who lives in Los Angeles or Miami, you won't be able to ski every day, so a muscular-endurance activity for your legs cannot be done on the slopes—it must be done in the gym or at home.

Isolating the Joint Action

You can seldom isolate just one muscle, but you can isolate a joint action. For example, flexing the biceps is a single-joint action, even though two other muscles are working along with the biceps muscle. When you lift a barbell in a curl, you are also exercising the muscles in the front of the forearms and hands; they are contracting because they are gripping the bar.

1. Neck

Neck strength is important in activities where your head may take a blow from an opponent or from a fall, such as in football, soccer, wrestling, and gymnastics.

Some gyms have head harnesses on which the lifter can hang weights and lift them with the head. And there are some machines, usually isokinetic, that have neck-strength stations. But the simplest way to gain neck strength is to use your own arm strength.

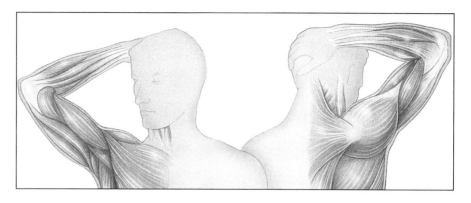

1A. Back of the neck

With your hands behind your head and your head forward, push your head back, resisting with your arms as much as possible. (But let your head win the battle!)

1B. Front of the neck

Place your hands on your forehead and tilt your head back. Bring your head forward as far as it will go.

Back of neck (1A)

Front of neck (1B)

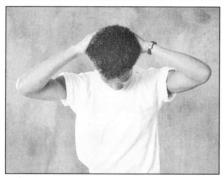 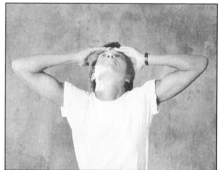

Side of neck (1C)

Rotary neck (1D)

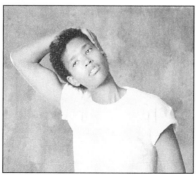 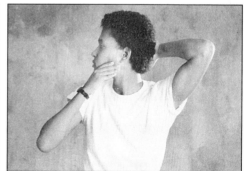

1C. Side of neck

Place your right hand on the right side of your head, allow your head to tilt all the way to the left, then force it right against the resistance of your right arm and hand. Repeat the exercise to the left side.

1D. Rotary neck

Place your right hand against your right temple or jaw and twist your head until you are looking over your right shoulder. Repeat with left hand at left temple or jaw until looking over your left shoulder.

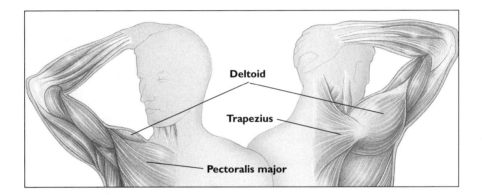

2. Shoulders

Upper Shoulders

The upper shoulders are involved in every lifting, throwing, and hitting activity. They are, therefore, very important in athletic competition.

2A. Deltolds: front of shoulders (standing forward raise)

The standing forward arm raise is for runners or those pitching underhand. Stand with dumbbells in each hand and raise the weight forward as high as possible. Runners should hold the palms inward; softball pitchers should hold them forward. This exercise can be done with both arms working at the same time, or you can alternate them.

Standing forward raise (2A)

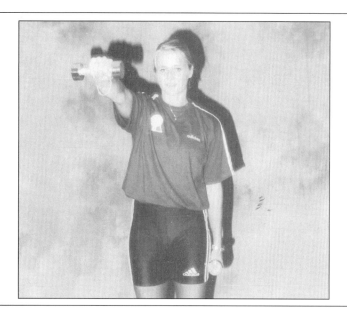

Standing fly (2B)

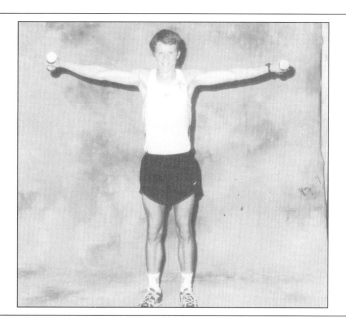

2B. Deltoids: top of shoulders (standing lateral raise or "fly")

While standing with dumbbells in your hands and at your side, lift the dumbbells sideways directly overhead with the backs of your hands staying on top of the dumbbells. (If you turn your hands palms up, you will be able to lift more

Bent flys (2C)

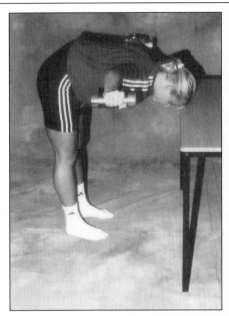 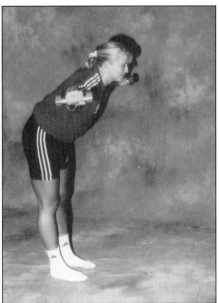

weight because you will be allowing the upper chest muscles ("pecs") to join in the work. You probably don't want this.)

This exercise also works the upper part of the trapezius—the large muscle in the middle of your upper back.

2C. Deltolds: back of shoulders (bent lateral raise or "fly")

While bent at a 90-degree angle at your waist, and with your head on a table or against a wall to reduce the pressure on the lower spinal discs, raise the dumbbells from directly below the shoulders as far up as they will go to your side. Keep your arms straight. This exercise can also be done without the full 90-degree bend.

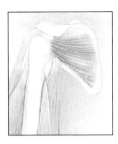

Rotator Cuff

The rotator cuff muscles turn the upper arm in the shoulder socket. These very important muscles come into play in most throwing and hitting actions. They are particularly important in throwing a baseball, serving or spiking a volleyball, or hitting a golf ball. Because they are quite small, they are often injured. They should, therefore, be exercised both for maximum strength and for injury prevention.

2D. Rotator cuff on back

While lying on your back on a mat or bench, hold a dumbbell with your elbow at a 90-degree angle to your side. Bring the dumbbell to a vertical position, then continue the action until the weight is touching your abdomen. Return to the starting position. This exercise will work two different actions of the rotator cuff muscles.

Rotator cuff on back (2D)

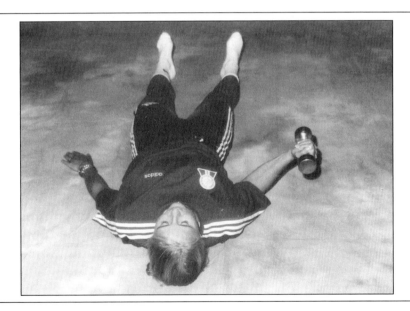

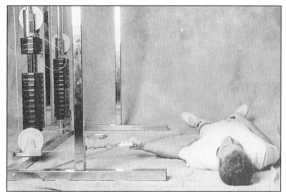
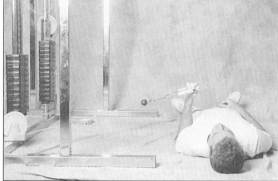

Rotator cuff on pulley (2E)

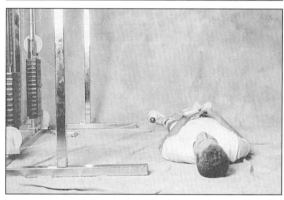

2E. Rotator cuff on pulley

Lie on the floor with your left side near the lower pulley of a machine, your left elbow next to your hip and flexed at 90 degrees, and your left hand on the handle. Pull the handle across your body by rotating your upper arm and keeping the elbow flexed.

From the same position, take the handle in your right hand and pull the handle across your body.

Change to sitting with your right side to the machine and work each exercise again.

The pulleys give you better resistance than the dumbbell exercise illustrated in 2D.

2F. Bent dumbbell pull-back

While standing, bent at the waist and with a dumbbell in each hand, pull the weights back toward your waist and turn them to the inside.

Bent rotator cuff exercises (2F)

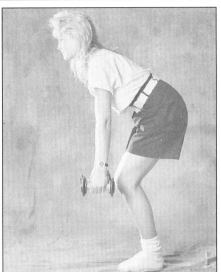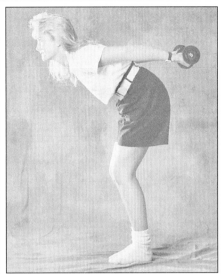

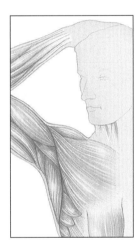

3. Chest

Upper Chest

The upper chest muscles are used in any pushing or throwing action.

3A. Supine lateral raise or "fly"

The front of the deltoids will work with the upper part of the chest muscle (the clavicular portion of the pectorals major). If the exercise is done flat on your back (the supine position), the pectorals will do more of the work. If you are on an incline with your head high, the deltoids will do more of the work.

Free weights (dumbbells) lend themselves well to this type of shoulder muscle isolation. While lying on your back, with a dumbbell in each hand, allow the

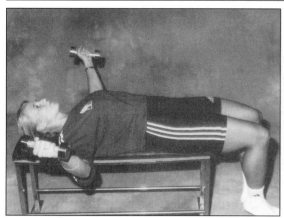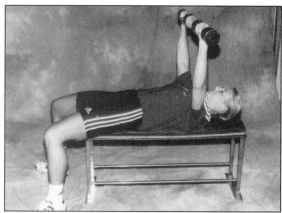

Supine fly (3A)

weights to come at least to the level of your body, then raise them with slightly flexed arms until your arms are vertical.

To add flexibility, you can do the exercises on a narrow bench and let the dumbbells come down past your body before lifting them. For this exercise, you will have to reduce the weight of the dumbbells a bit.

Lower Chest

The lower chest muscles are used in pulling yourself upward, such as in swimming or gymnastics. Working the lower chest muscles requires that you bring

Lateral raise in incline position (3A)

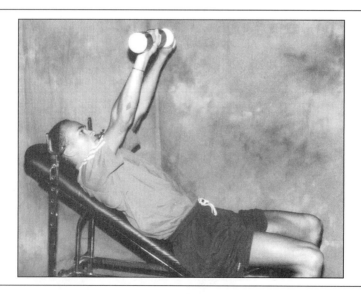

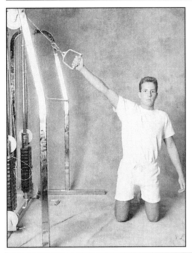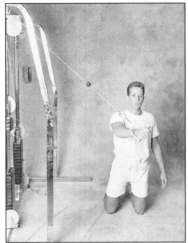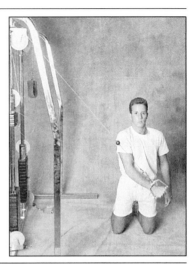

Lower chest exercise on
pulley (3B)

your arm toward your hips while you are working against resistance. This
means that for best results, you will either have to be on a steep incline with
your head down, called the *decline position*, or work with overhead pulleys.

3B. Lower chest exercise on pulley

With pulleys, start with your arm at about a 45-degree angle from the vertical,
then pull the resistance across your body—in front of your shoulders—finishing
at your opposite hip. This exercise will emphasize the lower part of your chest
(sternal portion of the pectoralis major—the part that attaches to the sternum,
or breast bone), but it also works the upper chest (clavicular portion—the part
that attaches to your clavicle, or collar bone).

3C. Sideways straight-arm lat pull-down on pulley

This pulley exercise works your lower chest with your *lats* (latissimus dorsi)
muscle. Facing sideways to the pulley, with your arm overhead, pull down the
handle until your arm is at your side.

3D. Lateral raise or "fly" in decline position

Do a decline lateral raise in which your head is lower than your torso while you
are on an incline board.

Sideways pull-down on pulley (3C)

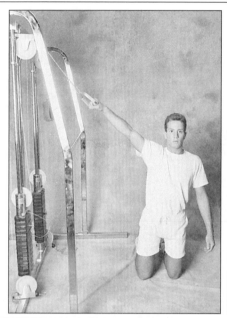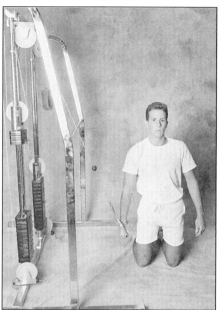

Lateral raise in decline position (3D)

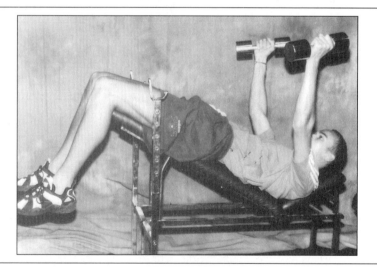

4. Upper Back

The upper and middle back muscles are important for good posture—they keep our shoulders back. They also assist in any pulling action, so are important in swimming and cross-country skiing.

For the top of your back (the upper part of your trapezius), you can use the same exercise that develops the top of the shoulders (standing lateral raise—see exercise 2B).

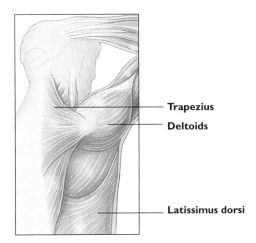

Trapezius

Deltoids

Latissimus dorsi

4A. Standing shoulder shrug

While standing, hold a barbell in front of you with your arms straight; then just lift your shoulders up without bending your arms. The trapezius muscle is quite strong, so a lot of weight can be handled in this exercise. This exercise can be done with a barbell or on a machine.

Standing shoulder shrug (4A)

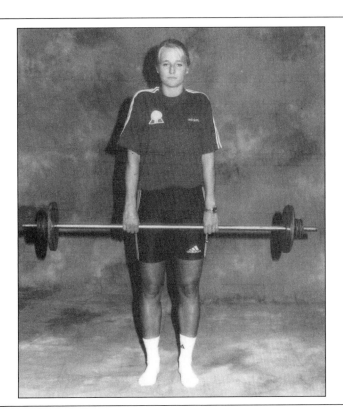

Bent shrug (4B)

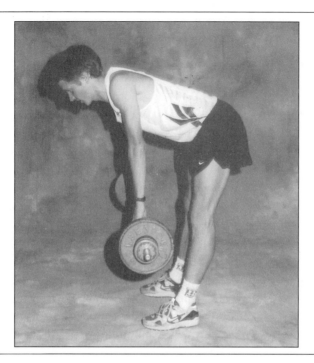

For the middle part of the trapezius, the same exercise that works the back of the deltoids (bent lateral raise) will do (see exercise 3C).

4B. Bent shrug

Bent shrugs will also develop this muscle action. In a bent position, with your head braced on a waist-high table or against a wall, and while holding a barbell at arm's length straight down, shrug your shoulders. (Don't flex your elbows.) Because of the potential strain on the discs of your lower back, this exercise is not often recommended.

4C. Straight-arm pull-down on lat machine

The lower part of your upper back (lower trapezius and latissimus dorsi) is best developed by pulling down on a pulley. Face the machine, and with your arms straight, pull down until you have pulled the bar to your hips. This will also work one head of the triceps muscle. Since your arms will start at about a 30-degree angle from the vertical, you will get most of your strength gain in the area in which you are working the muscle. If you want to gain strength in the top 30 degrees of the pull, either face away from the machine and start your pull with your arms directly overhead, or do pull-overs on the bench.

There are some machines that allow you to sit while you perform this exercise.

Straight-arm pull-down on lat machine

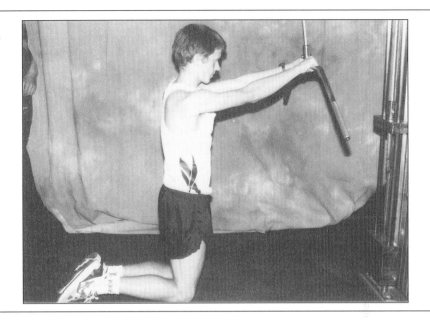

4D. Bent-arm pull-over

Bent-arm pull-overs increase the range of motion in which your muscles gain strength, because the weight starts at a lower position. You can use either a barbell or a machine for this exercise.

   Standing or kneeling sideways to a high pulley, pull the handle directly to the side of your thigh.

   The previously mentioned side pull-down for the lower chest will also work the lower part of your upper back (see exercise 3C).

Bent-arm pull-over (4D)

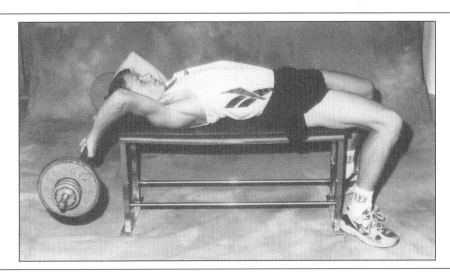

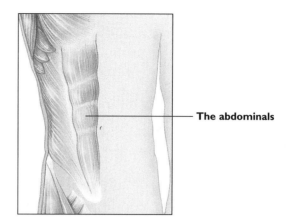

The abdominals

5. Abdominals

Most people are aware of how important it is to have abdominal strength. For one thing, it helps to keep our bellies tucked in for better posture. In addition, the abdominals help to stabilize the hips, which is essential for every athletic action that involves the hip joints, including running, jumping, swimming, gymnastics, and skiing. In fact, the abdominals, along with the lower back, are the two most important areas for strength in our bodies.

To isolate your abdominals, you should flex your knees as much as possible so that the muscles that flex the hip joint (bringing the thighs forward and upward) will not work as well. You should also keep your hips (your belt) on the mat when doing an abdominal exercise. Whenever your hips are pulled off the mat or bench, your hip flexors are working. This is particularly harmful for girls and women, who often have an excessive curvature in their lower backs. (This curvature places a higher pressure on the outside of the discs in the lower back region and can cause many problems as a person grows older.)

The reason hip flexion exercises can increase the curvature of the spine is that there are some muscles deep inside the pelvis that connect the lower back bones to the thigh bone. As they get stronger, they pull in on the lower spine and increase the curvature. You will often see this extreme lower back curve (technically called lordosis) in female gymnasts.

5A. Abdominal curl-up

Abdominal curl-ups are done by lying on the floor or on a bench with your knees bent and your hands on your chest or shoulders. (Some authorities believe that having the hands behind the head might increase the stress on the neck area, which is undesirable.) Curl your shoulders forward until your hips are about to leave the floor. Usually you will be able to touch your elbows to your thighs. A normal range of motion for abdominals is under 40 degrees. Keep your head up. Looking at the ceiling is a good idea. These can also be done on a machine.

Abdominal curl-up (5A)

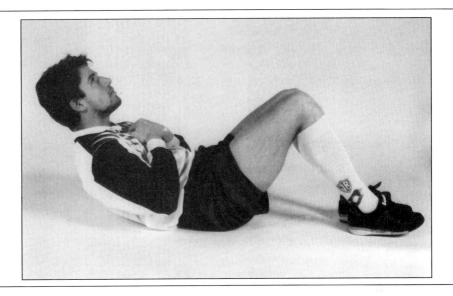

If you do the curl-ups on an inclined board with your head lower than your feet, you will increase the resistance you are lifting. If you are working for strength, you should hold weight plates on your chest in order to increase the resistance. But most people are looking for muscular endurance, to help hold their tummies in longer. If this is what you want, just do many repetitions. Herschel Walker, when playing professional football, did 3,500 repetitions daily.

Some people are not sufficiently strong to do this exercise correctly. In this case, it should be modified as follows: Grab the back of your thighs with your hands, and pull yourself up to the proper position. When this becomes easy, use only one hand on one thigh to help you curl up. Soon you will be able to do the exercise without using your hands to assist you. The exercise is easier with your hands on your hips, harder with your hands on your chest, and most difficult with your hands behind your head.

In a similar exercise, called the *abdominal crunch*, you lie flat on your back, then bring your knees and shoulders upward at the same time.

5B. Abdominal side sit-up

Side sit-ups are done to strengthen the muscles on the side of the abdominal area (the obliques). For this exercise, most people will have to have their feet held down. (They can be hooked under a barbell.) Lift your shoulders from the mat or bench. This exercise not only works the abdominal oblique muscles, but also the muscles on one side of your lower back and the rectus abdominis on the side to which you are bending.

5C. Rotary abdominal exercise

These can be done on a machine or by twisting the torso while doing a curl-up. Touch the left elbow to the right knee; then on the next curl-up, touch the right elbow to the left knee.

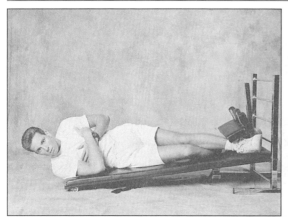 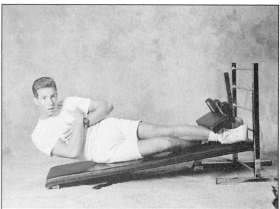

Side sit-ups (5B)

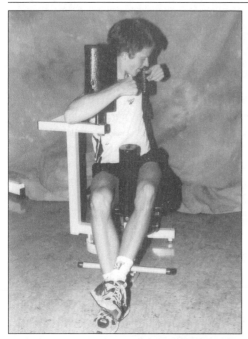 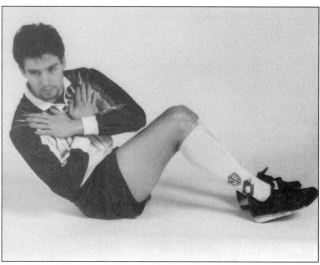

Rotary abdominal exercises (5C)

✓ *Checklist for Abdominal Exercises*

1. Flex your knees so that your hip flexors cannot contract effectively.
2. If your hips leave the bench or incline board, your hip flexors are contracting.
3. Think of yourself as curling up rather than sitting up.

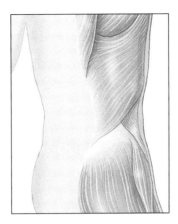

6. Lower Back

Exercises for the lower back are probably the most important for the average person to do, because lower back injuries, especially muscle pulls, are so common. They are often neglected, however, possibly because these muscles are less noticeable than many other muscles in our bodies.

The lower back muscles are particularly important in weight lifting, football, swimming, and skiing. And, of course, they are essential in maintaining good posture, because they are the muscles that hold our chests up by rotating our rib cages. They pull the back of the rib cage down, which raises the front of the rib cage and the chest.

6A. Back extension

Back extensions can be done on the floor. Just lie face down and raise your shoulders and knees slightly off the floor. Current thinking is that the back should not be hyperextended (greatly arched).

6B. Back extension using a Roman chair

In a gym there may be a *Roman chair* available, which will allow for a greater range of motion than the simple back extension of 6A. Put your hips on the small saddle, hook your feet under a bar, bend forward at the waist about 30 degrees, then straighten your back.

If you desire strength, hold weight plates or a dumbbell behind your head. If you want muscular endurance, just do as many reps as you can.

6C. Dead-lift

The dead-lift is a commonly used exercise for the lower back. Stand with your knees slightly flexed. With the barbell on the floor, grip the bar with your palms toward your body. While keeping your back straight and head up, straighten up to the standing position.

Back extension (6B)

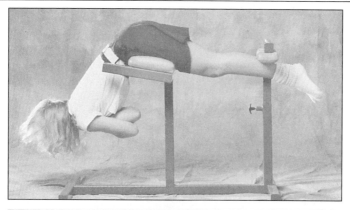

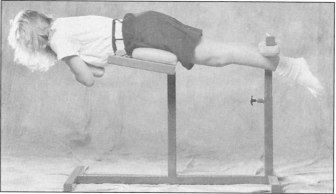

The problem with this exercise is that it may place excess stress on the inside edges of the discs of the lower spine. The stress could weaken them. Also, the weight being lifted is at its maximum while the pressure on the discs is at its maximum. In addition, the amount of force that your muscles are required to exert reduces during the exercise. By the time your back has moved through 30 degrees of motion, your muscles are lifting only 50 percent as much weight as they did when the weight was first being lifted from the floor.

6D. Dead-lift from back of shoulders

This so-called "good-morning" exercise is similar to the dead-lift, but the weight is carried on the back of the shoulders. The waist is allowed to bend forward until reaching a 90-degree angle, then is straightened back up to the standing position. This commonly done exercise is not recommended for most people.

Dead-lift from back of shoulders (6D)

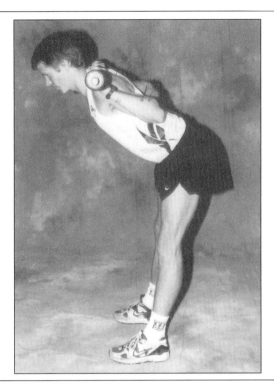

Hip flexors

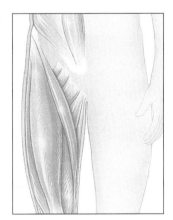

7. Hip Flexors

The hip-flexor muscles bring our thighs forward, so they are essential in any running or jumping activity. As previously mentioned, though, hip-flexion exercises might be harmful for some people, especially women. However, many people need strength in the hip-flexor muscles—including gymnasts, dancers, and anyone who needs to run fast.

For those susceptible to an excessive lower back curvature, special precautions should be taken. They should keep the connective tissue in their lower backs flexible by doing toe-touching exercises. They should also keep their abdominals strong to reduce the tendency of the front of the hips to drop forward, which increases the curve of the lower spine.

Hip flexors are exercised when the thigh is brought forward. This can be done several ways: hanging or standing, without weights, with a weighted boot, or with an ankle attachment to a pulley on a machine.

7A. Knees to chest on high bar

While hanging from a high bar, bring your legs forward with your knees bent. Touch your knees to your chest.

7B. Legs forward on high bar

While hanging from the high bar, bring your legs forward without bending your knees.

7C. Leg raise (hip flexion) on pulley

Using the lower pulley of a weight machine, hook your ankle into a handle, or use an ankle strap to secure your ankle to the pulley. Raise your leg straight forward.

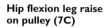

Hip flexion leg raise on pulley (7C)

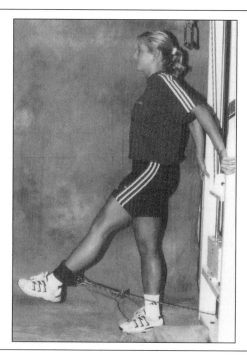

Standing leg lift (7D)

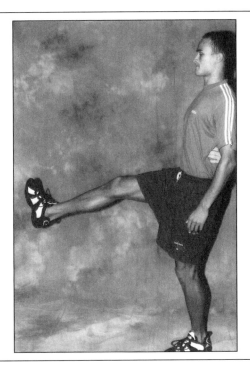

7D. Standing leg lift

While standing, with or without weight boots, brace yourself with your arms and lift one leg forward as high as it will go. Bring it up slowly.

7E. Leg lift in supine position

Lying on your back, lift one or both legs from the floor to the vertical position. Your abdominals will contract isometrically in this, as in all other hip-flexion exercises.

Leg lift in supine position (7E)

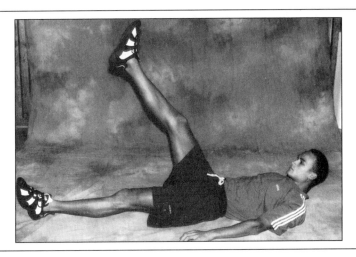

Knee extensors (8A, 8B)

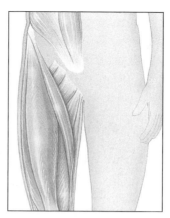

8. Knee Extensors (Leg Extension)

Extending the knee means straightening it. Knee extensors are, therefore, used in any running, jumping, or competitive weight-lifting activity.

Some of the major knee-extensor muscles also flex the hips. So the following exercises will also strengthen your hip flexors.

8A. Leg extension on machine

On the leg-extension machine, hook your feet under the padded bar, and straighten your leg. This exercise can also be done with a weighted boot.

Leg extension on machine (8A)

Keiser air resistance alternating leg extension machine (far right)
Photo courtesy Keiser

8B. Leg extension with partner

With a partner to provide resistance, sit on a table, and let your partner put both hands on your ankle. Straighten your leg while your partner gives you just enough resistance to allow you to make the movement.

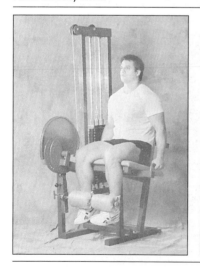
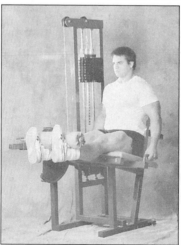
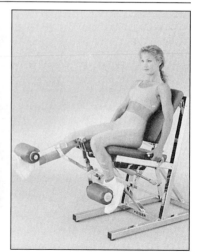

Leg extension with partner (8B)

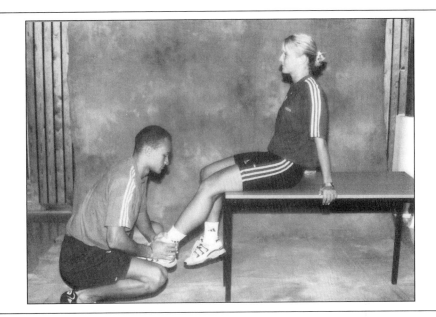

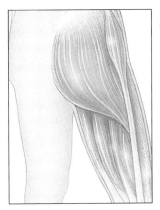

Hip (thigh) extensors (9A–C)

9. Hip (Thigh) Extensors

The hip-extensor muscles bring the thighs from a forward position back to a straight position (such as when you are standing). They will also bring the thighs farther back than straight, called *hyperextension*. The hip extensors are the muscles that supply power when you are running or jumping.

9A. Hip extension on machine

On a hip-extension machine, starting from a hip-flexed position, extend your thigh. On a pulley machine with ankle strap, face the machine, then extend and hyperextend the thigh.

Hip extension on pulley (9A)

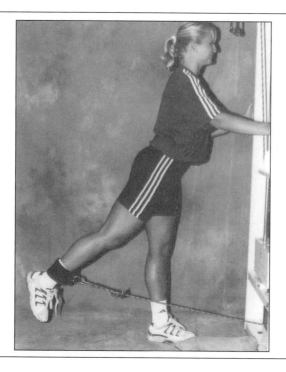

Hip extension with partner (9B)

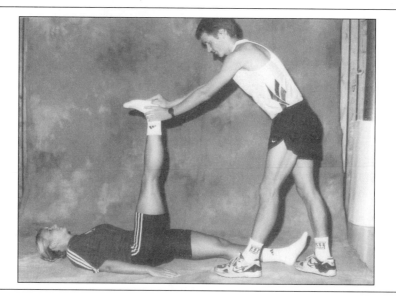

9B. Hip extension with partner

With a partner standing, lie on your back and bring your leg up. Let your partner hold the back of your ankle, then resist as you lower your leg to the floor.

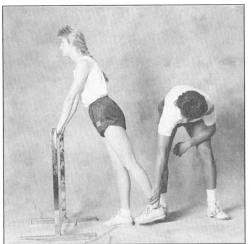
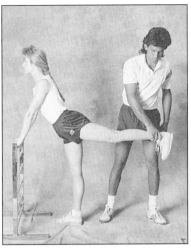

9C. Standing hip extension

While standing, bracing yourself for balance, bring one leg backward as far as you can. (This can be done with a partner.)

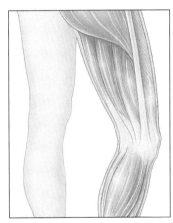

Knee flexors (10A, 10B)

10. Knee Flexors (Leg Curls)

The knee flexors bend the knee—decreasing the angle between the thigh and the lower leg. They generally work with the hip extensors, so are important in running. It is also essential that if the front of the thighs (the quadriceps or knee extensors) are strengthened, the knee flexors must also be strengthened.

10A. Leg curl (knee flexion) on machine

On a leg-extension machine, lie face down and hook your ankle under the bar. Flex your leg back at the knee joint. This exercise can also be done standing with a weighted boot.

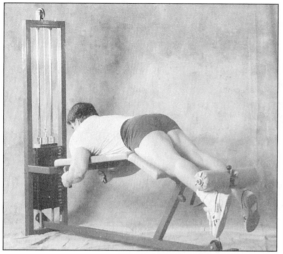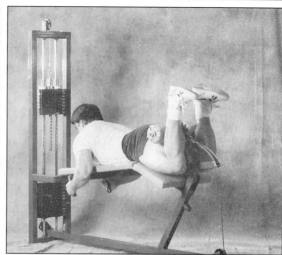

Knee flexion (leg curl) on machine (10A)

**Knee flex with part-
ner (10B)**

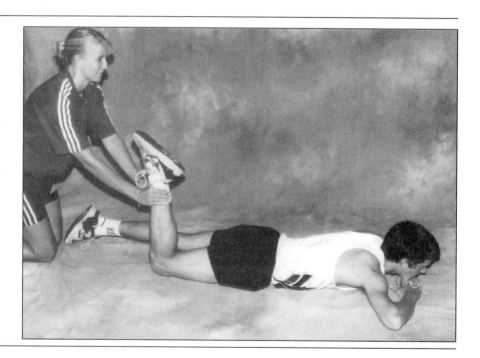

10B. Knee flexion with partner

Lie on the floor, and let your partner supply the resistance by putting his or her
hands on the back of your ankle as you flex your knee joint.

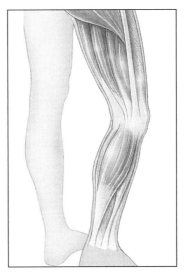

Knee flexors (10A, 10B)

11. Ankle Plantar Flexion

Ankle plantar flexion occurs when the sole of your foot moves closer to your calf muscle, as when you rise up on your toes. This is a key area for strength and power in running and jumping, for diving, and for pushing off on a turn in swimming.

11A. Calf exercise using barbell

Holding a barbell on your shoulders, rise up on your toes. This is better done with your toes on a riser board, or standing on a large weight plate, because your calf muscle will be gaining flexibility as you stretch down.

Calf muscle exercise (11A)

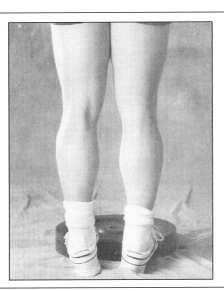
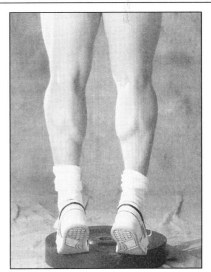

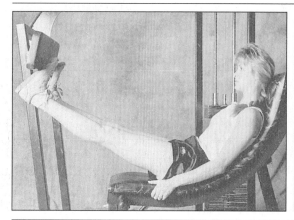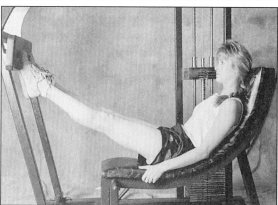

Calf muscle exercise on machine (11B)

11B. Calf exercise on machine

On a leg-extension machine or sled machine, with your legs straight, allow the weight to bring your ankles back, stretching your Achilles tendon. Then push the weight out with your calf muscles.

11C. Calf exercise using table

While holding a table for balance, rise up on one foot. This will give you the same resistance as holding a barbell equal to your body weight and doing the exercise with two legs. For example, if you weigh 150 pounds and hold a 150-

Calf muscle exercise using table (11C)

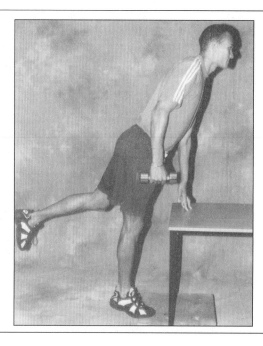

pound barbell, each of your calf muscles will be lifting 150 pounds. If you hold no weight but do the exercise with only one leg, the calf muscle will still be lifting 150 pounds.

By holding a dumbbell in your free hand and doing the exercise with one leg at a time, you get the same effect as adding double the amount to a barbell and doing the exercise with two legs.

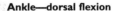

Ankle—dorsal flexion

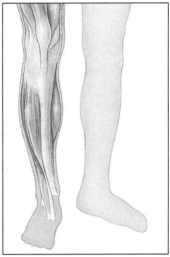

12. Other Ankle Exercises

You can also do ankle exercises to increase dorsal flexing strength (bringing the top of your foot forward) or turning the foot inward or outward. There are some weight machines which do this, but these exercises are more easily done with a partner or by giving yourself the resistance.

12A. Ankle joint: dorsal flexion

Dorsal flexion occurs when you bring the back (top) of the foot closer to the front of the knee. While pushing down on the top of your foot with your hand, allow the muscles in the front of your lower leg to bring your foot upward against the resistance of your hand.

This exercise can also be done while lying on your back on a leg-curl machine. Hook the toes under the pad and lift them toward your chest.

12B. Ankle joint: eversion

Eversion of the ankle joint occurs when you bring the outside of your foot upward. This action can be done to strengthen your ankle if you have had an ankle sprain. The damaged ligaments will take years to totally repair and

Dorsal flexion—ankle (12A)

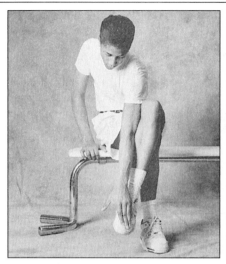
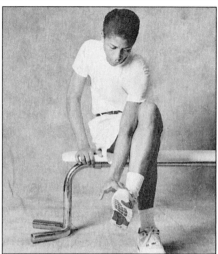

Ankle eversion (12B)

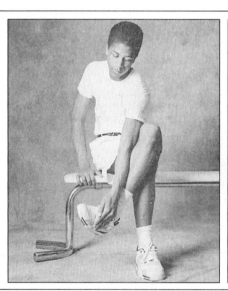
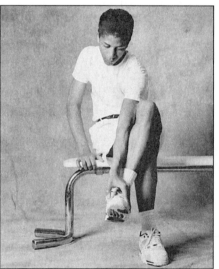

shrink, but by strengthening the muscles in the outside part of your lower leg, you may be able to prevent further ankle sprains.

To do this exercise, push down in the area of your little toe and bring your foot upward and outward against the pressure of your hand.

12C. Ankle joint: inversion

Inversion of the ankle occurs when the sole of the foot is brought inward. This action is not particularly useful. But if you have had an injury to those muscles

Ankle inversion (12C)

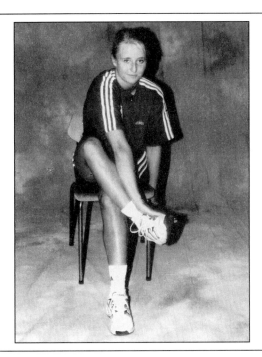

and want to strengthen them, you can simply put your hand under the foot, applying pressure to the outside edge of the sole of the foot, then turn the foot inward against that pressure.

Arm (elbow) flexors (13A–D)

Biceps

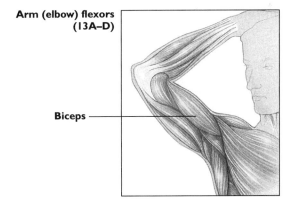

13. Arm (Elbow) Flexion

Arm flexion occurs when you bend at the elbow. The biceps curl is the exercise that strengthens this action. The curl can be done with a barbell, dumbbell, or a set of dumbbells. The biceps are used in football to tackle and to wrestle a ball away from another player (wide receiver or defensive back), in weight lifting to

Biceps curl with bar-bell (13A)

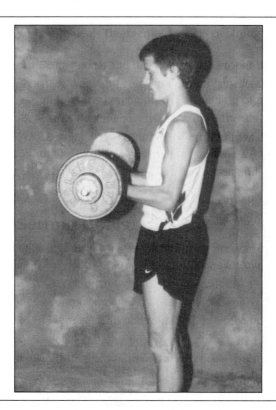

get the bar to shoulder height, in rowing to pull the oar, in basketball to rebound, in gymnastics for many actions, and in many other sports.

13A. Biceps curl using barbell

The barbell biceps curl is the most common biceps exercise. With the barbell in your hands (palms out) and your arms extended down, curl the barbell upward. The gripping of the bar will give you some isometric strength in the front of your forearms.

If you want additional strength in the back of your forearms, you can grip the bar with your palms facing inward at the start, called the *reverse grip*. This additional strength in the back of your forearms may be helpful if you are a tennis player or golfer.

13B. Alternating curls using dumbbell

Alternating dumbbell curls are done by curling one dumbbell, then the other. This exercise is really just a variation of the barbell curl previously mentioned.

Alternating curls with dumbbells (13B)

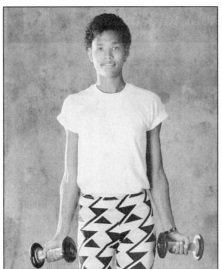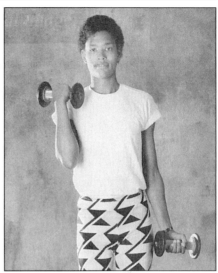

13C. Biceps curl in sitting position

Another biceps exercise is done in the sitting position while bracing your upper arm against your thigh when curling the dumbbell. (This eliminates "cheating" by swinging the weight.)

13D. Biceps curl on machine

On a weight machine, you can use the bench press station to curl, or you can use the lower pulleys.

Bicep curl—sitting (13C)

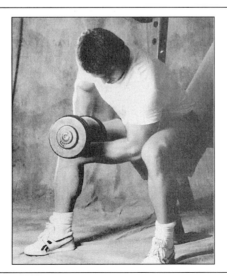

Bicep curl on machine (13D)

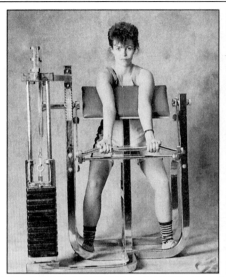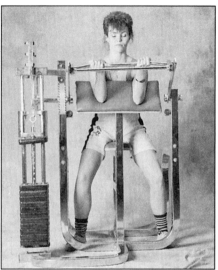

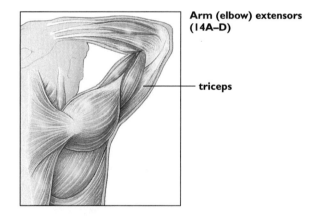

Arm (elbow) extensors (14A–D)

triceps

14. Arm (Elbow) Extension (Triceps Extension)

The triceps are used to straighten your arms. They are therefore used in pushing something away from the body and in throwing. In athletics they are used in football for pass-protection blocking and for hand shivers by defensive linemen; in weight lifting they help in the pressing action; in ice skating and dance they aid in lifting one's partner; in swimming they assist throughout the whole stroke; in gymnastics they are used in handstands; in baseball they are used to both throw and hit; in basketball they are used to shoot and pass; in tennis they are used in the serve; and in golf they assist in the downswing. In short, they are used a great deal.

Standing triceps extension (14A)

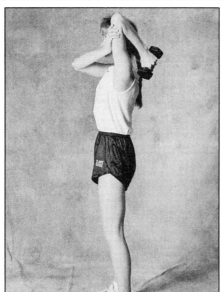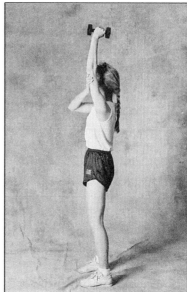

14A. Standing one-arm triceps extension

This is the best exercise for arm (elbow) extension. Start with the arm holding the dumbbell extended overhead. Steady that elbow with the other hand by holding just below the elbow on the extended arm. (This stops you from "cheating" by allowing other muscles to come into play.) Allow the dumbbell to lower as much as possible. (This gives maximum flexibility.) Then raise the dumbbell overhead for strength.

14B. Triceps push-down

On a weight machine, use the high-pulley station. Grip the bar, and with your elbows at your side, bring the bar down by straightening your arms—a triceps push-down. This exercise does not give as much flexibility as exercise 14A.

14C. Two-arm triceps extension

Some people like to exercise both triceps at the same time. If you prefer this, use either a dumbbell or a barbell, lower it behind your head, and extend it overhead.

The problem with this exercise is that it is almost impossible to do without bringing in other muscles that move the shoulder joint. Also, using a heavy barbell can pull you off balance—especially if your arms are perpendicular to the floor in the maximum stretching position.

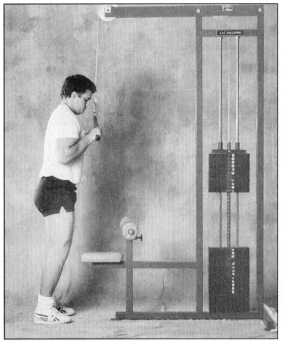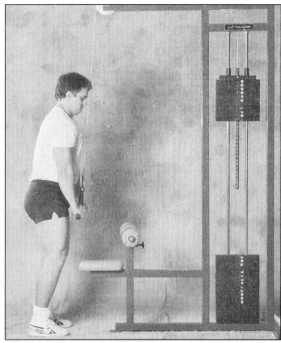

Triceps push-down on machine (14B)

14D. Triceps extension with manual resistance

To use your own muscles to give you resistance, flex one arm, then put the hand of the other arm against the wrist of the flexed arm. Straighten the arm while resisting with the other hand.

Triceps extension—manual resistance (14B)

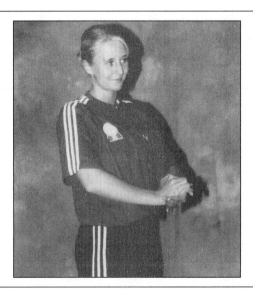

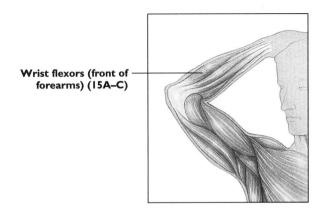

Wrist flexors (front of forearms) (15A–C)

15. Wrist Flexion (Front of Forearms)

The wrist flexors are used in any throwing or hitting motion. They put the curve on a curve ball and the "fast" in a fast ball, they bring the tennis racket upward in a serve, and they supply some of the power in the golf swing, the tennis forehand, and in hitting a baseball.

15A. Wrist curl using barbell or dumbbell

Sit down while straddling a bench. With a barbell or dumbbell in your hands (palms up), and the back of your forearms on the bench, let the weight hyper-extend your wrist, then flex your wrist forward. This exercise can also be done with a dumbbell exercising one wrist, then the other.

Wrist curl (15A)

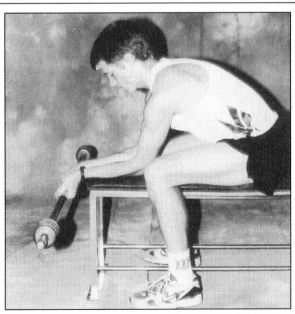

Wrist curl with manual resistance (15B)

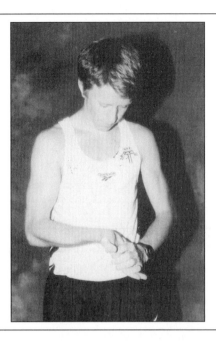

Some people will use a weight attached by a rope to a handle. The exerciser raises the weight by rolling the handle by alternate wrist movements. This is not good for maximum strength gain, but it is fine for bulk work or muscular endurance.

15B. Wrist curl with manual resistance

The wrist can also be strengthened by using your own hand as the resistance (on the palm of your exercising wrist), or by using a broom or pole as the resistance, lifting the broom with your palm facing up.

Wrist curl using broom (15C)

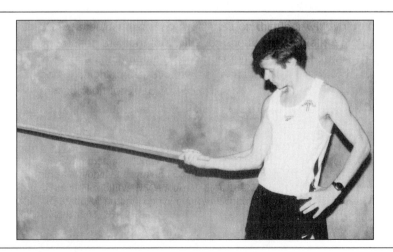

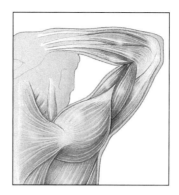

16. Wrist Extension (Back of Forearms)

The wrist extensors are important in stabilizing the wrist in any backhand action—in tennis, racquetball, or golf. They are also essential in weight-lifting competition because they tend to be the weakest link in the "cleaning" action that brings the bar from the floor to the chest.

16A. Reverse wrist curl using barbell or dumbbell

While sitting and straddling a bench (as in exercise 15A), with your hands grasping the barbell (palms down), let the barbell flex your wrists, then extend your wrists upward. This exercise will strengthen the back of your forearms. You will probably be able to use only about two-thirds of the weight that you were able to handle in the wrist-flexion exercise.

**Reverse wrist curl
(16A)**

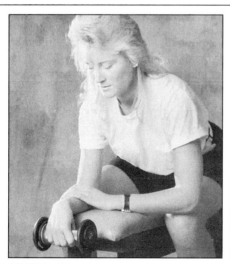
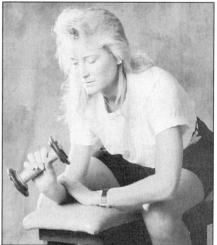

Reverse wrist curl with manual resistance (16B)

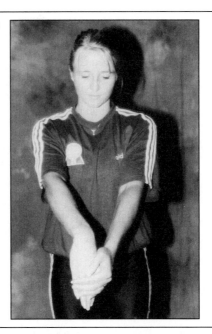

16B. Reverse wrist curl with manual resistance

You can also use your hand on the back of the other hand as resistance, or lift a broom or pole with your palm facing the ground.

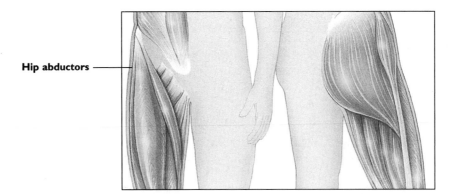

Hip abductors

17. Hip Abduction

Hip *abduction* means moving your leg sideways in a lateral plane. It uses the muscles on the outside of the hips, which are important to anyone who wants to move laterally while facing ahead. It is used by basketball players playing man-to-man defense, by football players (especially defensive linemen), by dancers, and by gymnasts. Golfers use it in developing the leg power of their swings.

Hip abduction on machine (17A)

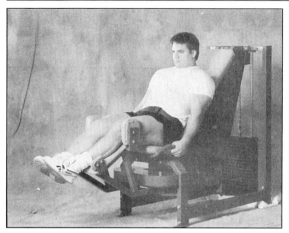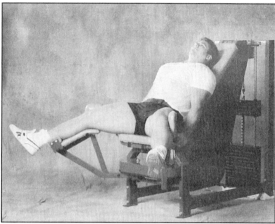

17A. Hip abduction on machine

If you have an abduction machine, just sit in the seat, hook your legs into the stirrups, and push both legs outward.

17B. Hip abduction with partner

Lie on your back with your partner holding the outside of your feet or lower legs. Push your legs apart as far as they will go, with your partner resisting.

Hip abduction with partner (17B)

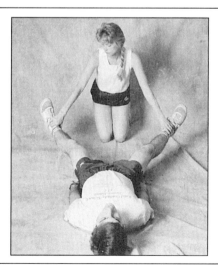

Hip abduction on pulley (17C)

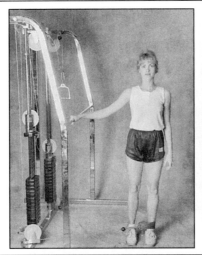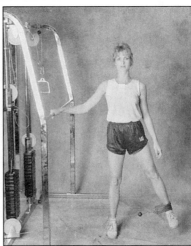

17C. Leg pull with pulley

On a machine, use the lower pulley. While standing sideways to the machine at the low pulley station, hook your foot into the handle (or use an ankle strap) and pull your leg away from the machine.

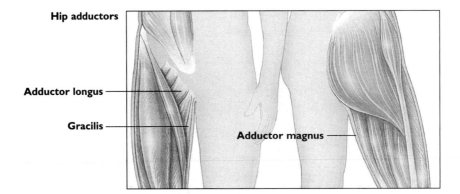

Hip adductors

Adductor longus

Gracilis

Adductor magnus

18. Hip Adduction

Hip-*adduction* exercises strengthen the muscles on the inside of the leg (the groin area). These muscles are used in moving laterally, so they are very important to swimmers doing the breast stroke.

18A. Hip adduction on machine

With an adduction machine, sit in the seat, put your legs on the proper part of the machine, and squeeze your legs together.

Hip adduction with partner (18B)

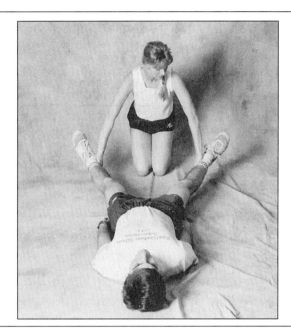

18B. Hip adduction with partner

Lie down with your legs spread, and have your partner put his or her hands on the inside of your knees or lower legs, giving you resistance as you squeeze your legs together.

Hip adduction on pulley (18C)

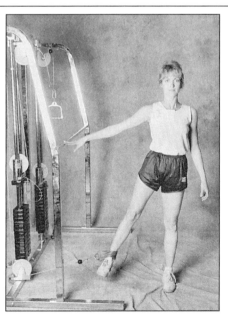 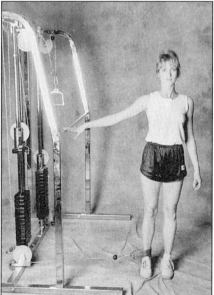

18C. Hip adduction with pulley

On a machine with a low pulley, while standing away from the machine and sideways to it, and with your foot in the ankle strap, squeeze your leg in toward your body, pulling the foot away from the machine.

Summary

1. One-joint exercises are an essential part of any strength-training program.
2. There is at least one exercise for every joint action.
3. The abdominal and lower back areas are extremely important areas to strengthen.
4. Many athletic events require strengthening of certain one-joint actions.

8 *Multiple-Joint Exercises*

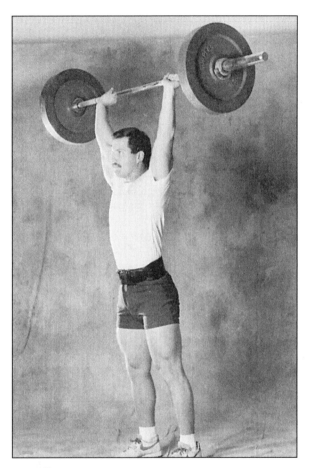

Outline

Multiple-Joint Exercises
Checklist for Safety
*Checklist for Loading and Unloading
    a Barbell*
Checklist for the Snatch
Summary

Many of the traditional bodybuilding exercises are multiple-joint exercises. Since people who use weights to train generally want either bulk or specific strength and power for an athletic activity, such exercises make sense, because they work two or more muscle groups at the same time. Even though one of the muscles involved may not be working to its maximum, at least it is working. A bench press (using upper chest, anterior deltoids, and triceps) or a lat pull-down (using biceps, lats, and lower chest) are examples.

Thus, multiple-joint exercises are a wise choice for developing bulk or for general conditioning. As total body strength is increased in a general conditioning program, the athlete can begin doing other exercises that are specific to the sport for which he or she is training. Some of these may be traditional multiple-joint exercises as well, although others may not. The athlete should analyze the actions of the sport and make the exercises approximate those actions.

Multiple-Joint Exercises

19. Bench Press

The bench-press action is used in actions such as passing a basketball, pass blocking in football, and defensive-line techniques. And, of course, it is a major lift for power lifters.

The bench press works the triceps, the front of the shoulders, and the upper chest muscles. If any of these muscles is weak, the lifter should do exercises that isolate the weaker muscles and strengthen them along with working on the bench press.

This press is done on a bench rather than on the floor, because your arms should be able to come below shoulder level for flexibility. Your grip should be wide enough so that when you lower the bar to your chest, your forearms should be perpendicular to the floor. If you want straight-ahead "pushing" strength, such as desired by football linemen, use the closer grip in which your

Bench press (19)

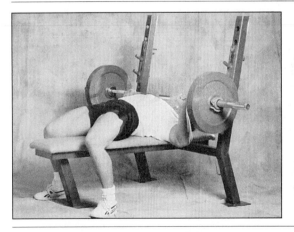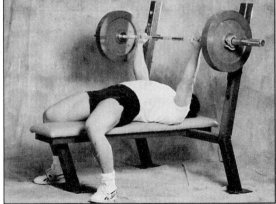

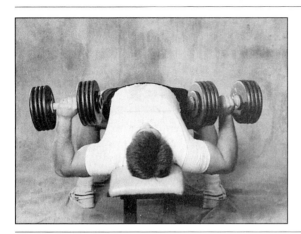 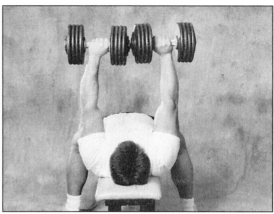

Dumbbell press

hands are directly above your shoulders. A wider grip will put more load on the muscles of the chest, while a grip with the hands closer will require more work from the triceps and deltoids.

Your back should remain on the bench throughout the exercise. If you arch, you will be able to lift a bit more weight because more of your lower pectorals will come into play. But this is considered "cheating."

Starting with the bar at arms' length and over your nose, slowly lower the bar to your chest, then push it upward. Be careful that you don't push it toward your feet, or you might lose control of it. The proper path of the bar is an arc from a position over the lifter's nose, lowered to the area of the nipples, then lifted over the nose. The bar should not go straight up from the chest, nor should it be bounced off the chest.

This exercise can be done with free weights using a rack and a spotter, or without a rack and with two spotters. The spotters are necessary to make certain that the lifter does not lose control of the weights, which may cause serious injury and even death. (Nearly all reported deaths related to strength training have occurred with boys doing bench presses alone and losing control of the weight, usually suffocating with the barbell on the neck. See Chapter 13 on injuries.)

✓ Checklist for Safety

1. Use a rack if one is available for all heavy lifts.
2. If no rack is available, use two spotters, one stationed at each end of the bar. (If only one spotter is available, the person should stand where he or she can best assist in controlling the weight. Usually this is behind the lifter.)

The bench press can also be done on a machine. The advantage of the machine is that it is safer. Also, on a machine your muscles do not have to balance the weights with other stabilizing muscles, since the balance is built into the machine. Some experts argue that the free weights force you to use other muscles than the primary muscles exercised, thereby stabilizing the joint. For example, in the bench press the primary movers are the chest and triceps muscles, but the deltoids, lats, and lower pectorals are all working to stabilize the lift so that the bar does not go too far towards your head or feet.

Dumbbells can also be pressed.

20. Incline Bench Press

The incline bench press works the front (anterior) deltoids more than the upper chest. It should be the favorite exercise of shot-putters. It is also important for football defensive linemen.

Select the proper angle for the incline bench—the angle at which you desire to work (45 degrees for a shot-putter)—and perform the press just as you did the supine bench press.

It can also be done with dumbbells.

21. Overhead (Military, or Shoulder) Barbell Press

This action is used in handstands in gymnastics, and in such events as ice skating and dance when the dancers lift their partners.

The overhead press is generally done standing, but many machines allow the lifter to sit, which decreases balance problems. If you are using this kind of

Incline bench press (20)

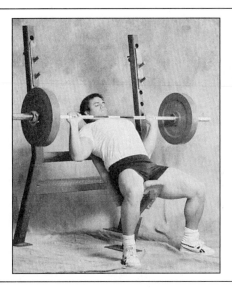 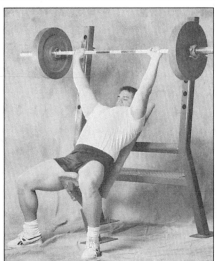

Dumbbell incline press (20)

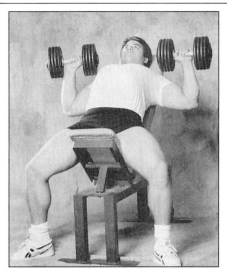 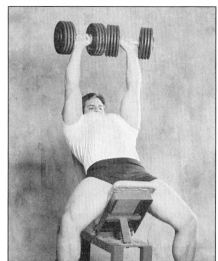

Standing overhead barbell press (21)

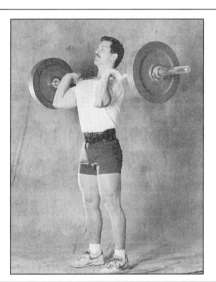 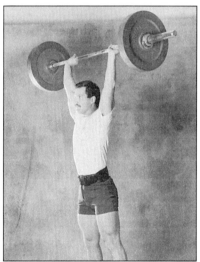

strength in an athletic activity, such as lifting a person, you should do it standing so that you can get used to balancing the weight with your whole body.

A variation of this press is the *push press*, in which the lifter flexes the knees to about 30 degrees, then forcefully extends the legs and pushes the weight upward.

The overhead press can also be done with dumbbells. The action can also be done with the weight being started behind the head.

Seated overhead dumbbell press (21)

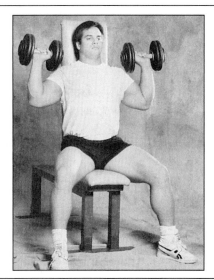 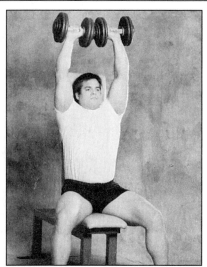

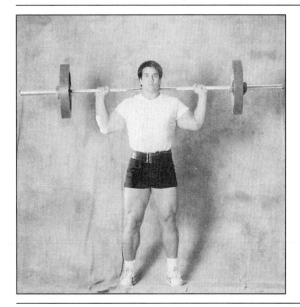 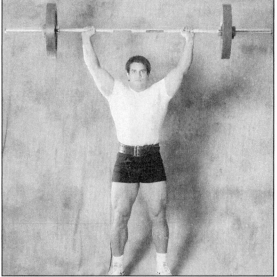

Shoulder press starting barbell behind the neck

When doing this press, be certain that you don't hyperextend your back. Such hyperextension can place great strain on the spinal discs in the rear of the vertebral column.

Checklist for Loading and Unloading a Barbell

1. Loading and unloading the weights is a major cause of finger injury to lifters who do not use the proper loading techniques.
2. Grip the weights firmly to avoid dropping them.
3. When loading the bar, be certain that the hollow part of the weight is on the inside. This makes it easier to grip the plate. It is important that the weights on both sides of the bar match (hollow side in), or the bar will be off balance.
4. Make certain that the bar is weighted correctly. If one side of the bar has heavier weights than the other, it will be significantly off balance and can result in an accident and possible injury to the lifter.
5. Collars should always be used to keep the weight plates secure and to prevent them from sliding and unbalancing the bar.

22. Lat Pull-Downs and Chin-Ups on a High Bar

Lat pull-downs and chin-ups work the biceps, lats, lower chest, and the muscles of the mid-back area. They are used in gymnastics, rope climbing, and climbing walls (a common military and police exercise).

For rope-climbing strength, you should grip the bar with your palms facing you. For strength to climb walls, your palms should be facing away from you.

On a lat machine you will have to kneel or sit under the pulley. Then grip the bar wide and pull it down to your chest, or behind your back.

Lat pull-down (22)

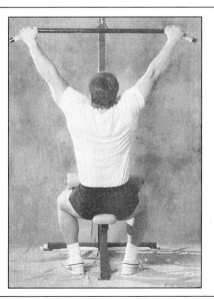 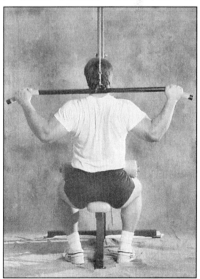

Squat (23)

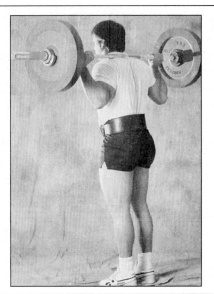
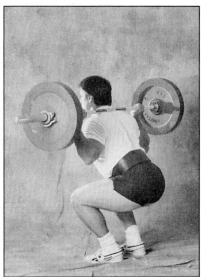

For chin-ups, grasp the high bar, using either the underbar or the overbar grip, and pull up until your chin is over the bar. You can add weights to your body if you want to increase the resistance.

23. Squat (Leg Press)

Squats, or leg presses, work the hip and knee extensors. These are necessary for nearly any running or jumping activity.

In performing a squat, make sure that the angle of your knee does not pass the 90-degree mark. At this point the ligaments that attach to the cartilage inside the knee are pulled back in the knee and act as fulcrums. The force of the weight downward on this fulcrum increases the stretch on the ligaments in the front of the knee and can stretch them too much—making the knee structurally weaker. In a *full squat*, the muscles at the back of the thighs and the calf muscles touch, and the fulcrum is moved further to the rear, causing great force to be exerted on the ligaments in the front of the knee.

Many weight lifters will do the squat to the point where the line of the top of the thighs is parallel with the ground. And Olympic lifters may go past that point, because it will be required in their competitive lifts.

23A. Squat in a squat rack

For maximum safety, squats should be done in the squat rack. In deciding how far down you will go in your squat, first determine why you want the strength. If you are a competitive weight lifter, you may wish to go past the 90-degree

Squat rack (23A)
Photo courtesy York
Barbell

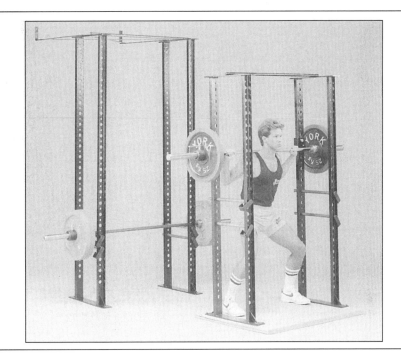

angle so that you can gain strength through a greater range of motion. But be aware that you may weaken the structure of your knee by stretching some of the ligaments. If you are a football lineman, you won't have to go past the 90-degree angle to develop the strength you need for that sport. If you are a high jumper or basketball player, you don't even have to go as far as 90 degrees—30 degrees may be far enough. Of course, if you are only bending your knees 30 degrees, you will be able to handle a great deal more weight than if you did a full squat. You should always start with a full range (90-degree) series, then you can do whatever other leg work you need to do.

When doing squats in the squat rack, be certain that the pins are set so that you cannot go too far down and damage your knees.

The most common positions for your feet are either shoulder width with the toes pointed straight ahead, or a wider-than-shoulder position with the toes pointed slightly outward. The feet should remain flat through the entire lift.

Cautions: Be certain to keep your back slightly arched and your head level or up to reduce pressure on the spinal discs. Don't let your torso bend too far forward. Also, don't let your knees get too far ahead of your toes. This would indicate that you are carrying too much weight forward, and you could lose your balance. It also increases the angle of the knee and can put harmful pressure on the ligaments. Furthermore, be careful not to bounce up from the squat position, because this also increases the strain on your knee ligaments.

During the squatting action, the bar should move up and down in a vertical path.

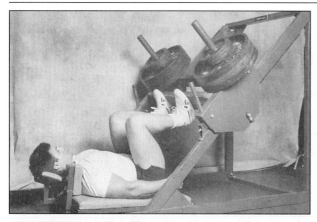

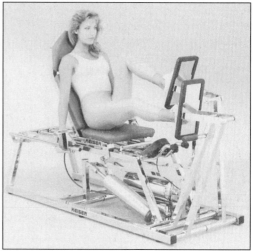

Keiser leg-extension machine can be used to simulate running
Photo courtesy Keiser

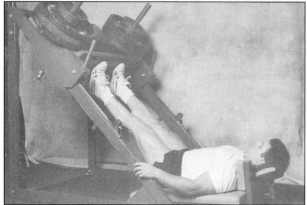

Leg press on machine (23B)

Two variations of the squat are the *front squat*, with the bar held on your chest, and the *hack squat*, with the bar held behind your back at the level of your buttocks.

23B. Leg press on machine

On the leg press machine, you have some built-in safety. By sitting down, you avoid the compressing force of the weight downward on your spinal discs.

As in the squat rack, you can finish your leg press on the machine with a toe push (ankle plantar flexion) to make the exercise more like a jump or a sprinting stride.

23C. One-legged squat using a table

If you don't have a full weight set and a squat rack and still want to do a squat exercise, you can do one-legged squats. Hold on to a table for balance, lift one foot off the floor, and squat with the other leg. This will give you the same effect as if you were carrying your body weight on a barbell.

Lunge (24)

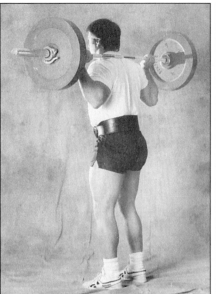 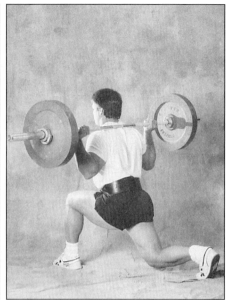

For example, if you weigh 150 pounds and do a one-legged squat, that is the same as doing a full squat holding a 150-pound barbell. This exercise is very valuable for people who are not consistent weight trainers but need good strength or muscular endurance for an event. It is a great pre-season and in-season exercise for skiers.

24. Lunge

This exercise works the same muscles as does the squat. With a barbell held on your shoulders behind your neck (or dumbbells held at your sides), take a step forward, and flex the forward leg as you settle into the lunge. Your knee should be no farther forward than your toes. Push yourself back up, and bring the forward foot back to the starting position. You may need two smaller steps to safely return to the starting position.

25. Upright Row

Upright rowing is an essential exercise for those who are training for Olympic lifting. The exercise works biceps, deltoids, and the upper trapezius.

The exercise is done standing. It can be done with a barbell, dumbbells, or on a machine with a low pulley. With the bar held next to your body at arm's length (palms facing your body), lift the bar to the level of your chin, always keeping the elbows higher than the bar.

Lunge (24)

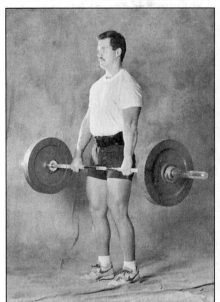 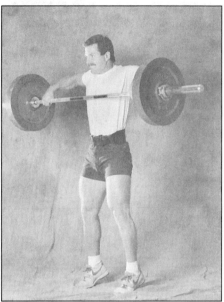

26. Bent Row

The bent-rowing exercise is important for those who like to row a boat or a racing shell. This exercise works the biceps, lats, and rear (posterior) deltoids. When it is done with a barbell, the back should be slightly arched and the hips should be flexed (the back flexed forward) about 60 degrees from the vertical. The knees should be slightly flexed.

Grip the bar with your palms facing your feet (a reverse grip), and lift the bar to the chest if you are more interested in developing the upper back. If you are more interested in developing the lats, lift the bar to your abdominal area.

The more you bend at the waist, the greater is the pressure on the lumbar spinal discs. The pressure has been calculated to be as high as 5,000 pounds per square inch for individuals lifting a heavy weight and bent forward (flexed) at 90 degrees. Consequently, some serious disc injuries have resulted from this exercise.

To reduce the strain on the lower back, you can use a dumbbell in one hand while placing your other hand on a bench to support your weight. On a machine you can use the low pulley. Either flex your torso forward, as with the barbell, or sit on the floor facing the pulley and pull the bar toward you.

27. Power Clean

The power clean is essential for competitive weight lifters, and is very useful for those wishing to develop full-body extension power. Football players fall

Bent row (26)

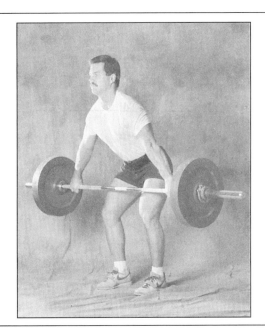

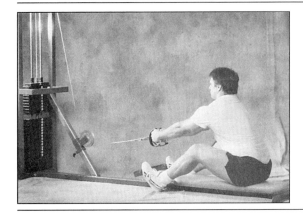
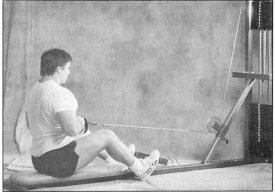

Row on machine

into this category. The exercise works the knee and hip extensors, the ankle plantar flexors, the lower back, the deltoids, the upper trapezius, and the biceps. Other muscles are involved to a lesser extent.

The barbell should be on the floor close to your feet. With your feet about shoulder width apart, bend forward with your back slightly arched, and grasp the bar with a wide grip and your palms facing toward you. Start the cleaning action with an explosive "jump" by straightening your hips, knees, and ankles. At the point where your legs are straightened, the bar will be moving fast. Use this velocity to help you pull the bar to chest level. At the top of the movement, bring your wrists back and push the elbows forward to allow the bar to settle

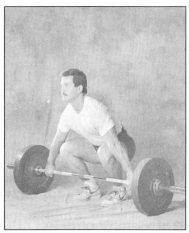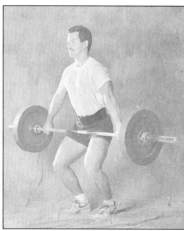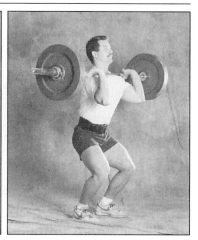

Power clean (27)

on the top of your chest—the *clean* position. At this point, flex your knees slightly to "catch" the weight. Then return the bar to the floor.

Another type of clean ends with the *high pull*, in which you lift the bar as high as possible, then return it to the floor without "catching" it.

The *hang clean* is often used to teach the power clean. It can also be used for those with weak or injured knees or backs. In this exercise, the barbell is dead-lifted to the waist. From this point it is raised to the clean position.

Power snatch (28)

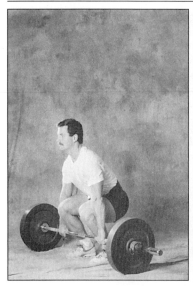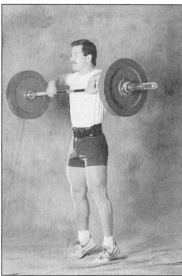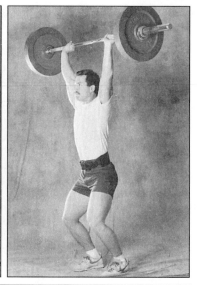

28. Power Snatch

The power snatch starts just as the clean, but you pull the bar above shoulder
level as high as possible. At the point where the bar is as high as it can be lifted, flex your knees and lock your arms under the bar. (Do not do this exercise
without knowledgeable supervision.)

This lift is done with a very wide grip and with lighter weights than the
power clean. The most common mistakes are letting the bar move too far forward—away from the body—or letting the elbows drop just as one is complet-
ing the pull and making a "hop" under the bar.

 *Checklist for the Snatch (for those
interested in Olympic-style lifting)*

1. Take a shoulder-width or narrower stance.
2. Squat down and grasp the bar very wide, using a hook grip (pinning your
   thumbs to the bar with your index fingers). This grip is important in overcom-
   ing the bar's inertia during the strong "second pull."
3. Keep your back flat at about a 45-degree angle to the floor.
4. Keep your shoulders well in front of the bar.
5. Lift the bar upward using only your legs. (Your back is at about the same angle
   to the floor as in the beginning position.)
6. Keep the bar close to your shins, and keep your shoulders over the bar. This
   will keep you in an effective position for the second pull.
8. As the bar passes your knees, re-flex the knees. (This is called the scoop or the
   double knee bend.)
9. Pull the bar upward and move under the bar quickly. This is a major key to
   effective lifting.
10. Quickly move to the squat position as the bar is extended (locked out) over-
    head.
11. Move to the standing position quickly, as the bar is still moving upward from
    the pull.
12. Hold motionless until the official signals that the lift is good, then return the bar
    to the floor while controlling it.

Summary

1. Multiple-joint exercises are the foundation for most strength-training programs.
2. The major types of multiple-joint exercises include:
   - Presses, both overhead (military) and bench
   - Pulling exercises, such as lat pull-downs, rowing, cleans, and snatches
   - Leg presses, such as squats and lunges

9

Exercises for Special Interests–Posture and Sports

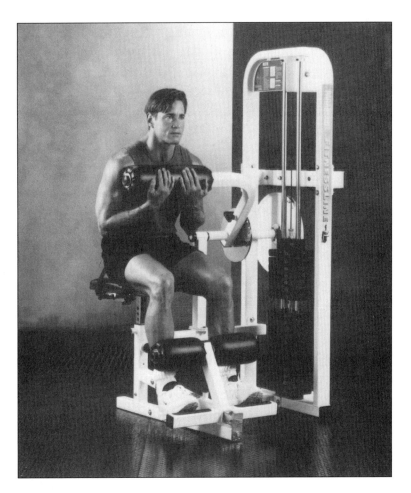

Outline

Exercises for Better Posture
Checklist for Posture
Exercises for Better Athletic Performance
The Specific Programs
Checklist for the Clean and Jerk
Checklist for General Muscle Strength
Summary

As has been mentioned, many areas of our lives can profit from greater strength or flexibility. Consider, for example, the benefits of good posture: looking more fit, having your clothes fit better, and enjoying increased health due to your internal organs being held in their proper places by tight abdominal muscles. Also, performance in any athletic activity will be enhanced by greater strength and flexibility.

Exercises for Better Posture

Better posture is achieved by stretching the front of your body and strengthening the muscles in the back. Assuming that you do not have structural abnormalities, the following postural problems can be helped.

Pot Belly

A pot belly can develop from drinking too much beer or from too much sitting. One cause of pot belly is tightened connective tissue (ligaments) in the lower part of the hip where it connects to the upper thigh bone. When these tissues are not stretched often, they become tight and pull the hip bone forward.

Left: **Pot belly and forward head hip stretch**
Right: **Hip stretch**

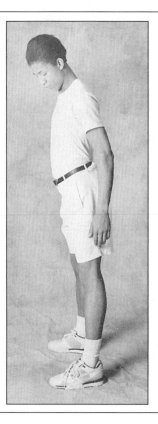
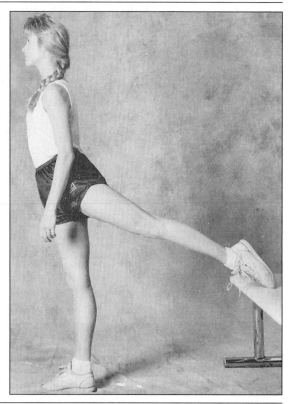

**Rounded shoulders
(left)**

**Shoulder stretch
(right)**

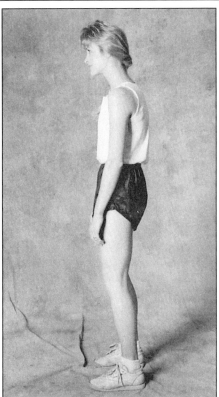 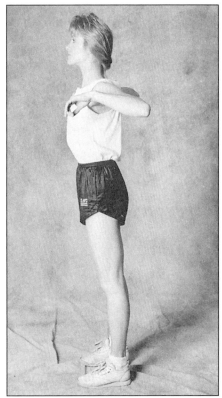

Stretching the hip flexors can bring back the flexibility of this joint. One simple way to stretch is to step forward with your left foot 3 to 4 feet. With your torso erect, tighten your abdominal muscles and push your hips forward. You can also put your foot behind you on a bench, then tighten your abdominals. You should feel the stretch in the lower front part of your right hip.

Round Shoulders

If your shoulders are rounded (a very common problem, especially for heavily muscled men and heavy-breasted women), you will need some stretching. While sitting or standing, you can pull your arms backward until you feel the stretch in your upper chest. Another exercise is done lying on a narrow bench. Take very light weights, 1 to 5 pounds, and with your arms straight, let the weights pull your arms down below your shoulders. Then try to pull them even farther down by contracting your upper back muscles. (Don't use heavy weights, because your chest muscles will fight to hold the weights, and you won't get as much stretch.)

Checklist for Posture

1. Do back extensions to develop the strength to rotate the lower rear part of your rib cage downward. This will lift the front top part of your ribs and "raise" your chest.
2. Do abdominal curl-ups to help pull the front of the hips upward and flatten your abdominals.
3. Do hip hyperextension stretches so that the connective tissue in the lower front of the hip joint is sufficiently flexible to allow you to raise the front of your hips.
4. Stretch the front of your shoulder girdle (the deltoids and pectorals) to reduce the chances of developing rounded shoulders through tight connective tissue.
5. Strengthen the rear part of your shoulder girdle (trapezium) through bent dumbbell raises or bent shrugs.
6. Stand tall, sit tall, and walk tall.

Sagging Chest

Lifting the chest is actually done with the small muscles in the lower back that pull down on the rib cage and thus "lift" the chest. Therefore, you should do lower back exercises to correct this postural problem.

Forward Head

A forward head is corrected by stretching the front of the neck and strengthening the back of the neck (exercise 1A in Chapter 7).

Overall Posture

For the necessary strength to allow you to hold a proper posture, see the following exercises in Chapter 7.
- To pull back rounded shoulders: 2C.
- To pull up a sagging chest: 6A and 6B. Other lower back exercises may also help: 4B and 4C.
- To pull back a forward head: 1A and 4B.
- To pull hips up (which requires strong abdominal muscles): 5A.
- To rotate hips back, (which requires strong gluteals): 9A, 9B, and 9C. (These muscles are already so strong that you probably won't need much work here.)

Once you have stretched your connective tissue to allow your bones to align properly, and have strengthened your muscles to allow you to hold the proper alignment, you just need to develop the habit of "standing tall." Try it. Stand as tall as you can. You will notice that all the right things happen. Your abdominal muscles will tighten. So will your hip extensors (buttocks) and your lower back muscles. You will probably have to consciously pull your shoulders back. Those muscles don't tighten normally when you stand tall.

You can also walk tall and sit tall. You will find that proper posture will make your chest look larger and your belly look smaller. It will look like you've lost 10 pounds. Good posture is a habit.

Exercises for Better Athletic Performance

The idea that working with weights made people musclebound has been replaced by the truism that both strength and flexibility training are essential for every athlete.

Male athletes were the first to use resistance training. Shot-putters and discus throwers led the way. Football players followed, and soon every athlete, male and female, found that strength training could greatly increase athletic abilities.

The General Strength Program

Many college strength coaches believe that every athlete should do a series of general body exercises before beginning the specific exercises for the sport. (Time limitations may, however, require a reduction or elimination of all or some of these exercises.) A general body strength program could include:

- Squats
- Bench press
- Lat pull-downs
- Shoulder (military) press
- Clean
- Hip abduction and adduction
- Curl-ups
- Back extensions
- Triceps exercise
- Biceps curl
- Calf raises

The Specific Programs

Because each athletic activity is somewhat different, each requires a different combination of exercises in order to develop an athlete's potential to the maximum. For example, participants in track events, football, basketball, and dancing all need a great deal of leg strength, while swimmers and golfers need much less. However, the swimmers, golfers, and gymnasts require much more strength in the lower chest and shoulder areas, because their events compel the use of arm pull rather than leg extension.

While an overall strength program may be good for everyone, special exercises can be particularly beneficial to athletes with special interests. Abdominal and lower back strength, on the other hand, is useful in nearly every sport.

Following are many sports in which specific strength training can increase athletic potential. The exercises listed can be found in Chapters 7 and 8.

Archery requires a great deal of strength in the upper shoulders, upper back, arms, forearms, and hands. The archer should therefore work especially hard on those areas. See exercises 2A (standing forward raise), 2C (bent lateral raise) 4B (bent shrug), 13A, 13B, or 13C (biceps curls), 14A, 14B, or 14C (triceps extension), 15 (wrist flexion curls), 16 (reverse wrist curls).

Badminton players need wrist strength and quick feet. They should concentrate on exercises 2D, 2E, 2F (rotator cuff), 7 (hip flexor), 8 (knee extension), 9 (hip extension), 10 (knee flexion), 11 (ankle plantar flexion), 15 (wrist curls), 16 (reverse wrist curls), 17 (hip abduction), 18 (hip adduction).

Baseball players need exercises 2D, 2E, 2F (rotator cuff), 3A (supine dumbbell fly), 5 (abdominal curl-up), 14 (triceps extension), 15 (wrist curls), 16 (reverse wrist curls), 17 (hip abduction), and 18 (hip adduction).

Basketball players need leg strength and upper arm pushing strength for shooting and passing. They should do exercises 11 (ankle plantar flexion), 14 (triceps extension), 15 (wrist curls), 17 (hip abduction), 18 (hip adduction), 19 (bench press), 20 (incline bench press), 22 (lat pull-downs or chin-ups on high bar) for rebounding, and 23 (squats or leg extensions), or 24 (lunge).

Football players need exercises 1 (all neck exercises), 5A (abdominal curl-up), 6 (back extension), 11 (ankle plantar flexion), 17 (hip abduction), 18 (hip adduction), and 23 (leg presses or squats) or 24 (lunge). Each position may require additional exercises.

Offensive linemen and running backs should do exercises 19 (bench press) for pass protection and stiff arm, and 27 (power clean).

Quarterbacks should do exercises 2D (rotator cuff dumbbell rotation) or 2E (rotator cuff pulley exercise), 2F (rotator cuff dumbbell pull-back), 3A (supine dumbbell fly), 14 (triceps extension), and 15 (wrist curls).

Wide receivers and defensive backs should do exercises 13 (biceps curls), 15 (wrist curls), and 22 (lat pull-downs or chin-ups on high bar).

Defensive linemen and linebackers should do exercises 13 (biceps curls) for tackling, 14 (triceps extension), 19 (bench press), 20 (incline bench press), 22 (lat pull-downs or chin-ups on high bar) for tackling, and 27 (power clean).

Kickers should do exercises 7 (hip flexors—from high bar or on a machine), 8 (knee extensors on machine), 11 (ankle plantar flexion)—for punters and soccer-style place kickers, or 12A (ankle dorsal flexion)—for straight-ahead place kickers.

Golfers can profit by extra work on 2D (rotator cuff dumbbell rotation), 2E (rotator cuff pulley exercise), 2F (rotator cuff dumbbell pull-back), 3C (sideways straight-arm pull-down on pulley), 4C (straight-arm pull-down on lat machine—facing the machine), 5A (abdominal curl-up) and 5B (side sit-up), 15 (wrist curls), 16 (reverse wrist curls), 17 (hip abduction), and 18 (hip adduction).

Gymnasts can use exercises for every muscle group. Their vaulting and tumbling require great leg strength and power, while other events require all the upper body exercises. They can profit by extra work in 3C (sideways straight-arm pull-down on lat machine), 5 (abdominal curl-up), 7A and 7B (hip flexion on high bar), 11 (ankle plantar flexion), 15 (wrist curls), 21 (overhead [military] press), 22 (lat pull-downs on machine or chin-ups on high bar), and 23 (squats or leg presses).

Racquetball and handball players should emphasize 2A (standing forward raise), 2C (bent dumbbell raise), 2D (rotator cuff dumbbell raise), 2E (rotator cuff on pulley), 2F (rotator cuff dumbbell pull-back), 7 (hip flexors from high bar or on machine), 15 (wrist curls), 16 (reverse wrist curls), 17 (hip abduction), and 18 (hip adduction).

Soccer players can use extra leg work so they should emphasize exercises 7 (hip flexors from high bar or on machine), 8 (knee extensors on machine or with a partner), 9 (hip extensors on machine or with a partner), 10A (knee flexion on machine), 11 (ankle plantar flexion), 17 (hip abduction), 18 (hip adduction), and 23 (squat or leg extensions) or 24 (lunge).

Skiers should do extra work on exercises 2C (bent lateral dumbbell raise), 4C (straight-arm pull-down on lat machine), 5 (abdominal curl-up and side sit-up), 6 (back extension), 17 (hip abduction), and 18 (hip adduction); and particular work on 7 (hip flexors from high bar or on machine), 8 (knee extensors on leg machine or with manual resistance), and 23 (squat or leg press) or 24 (lunge).

Softball players should do the same exercises as baseball players, but pitchers should add exercise 2D (rotator cuff exercise on back), 2E (rotator cuff exercise on pulley), and 2F (bent dumbbell pull-back).

Swimmers and water polo players both use the primary swimming muscles exercised in 2D (rotator cuff exercise on back), 2E (rotator cuff exercise on pulley), 2F (bent dumbbell pull-back), 3C (sideways straight-arm pull-down on pulley), 4C (straight-arm pull-down facing machine—this is the most important), 13 (biceps curl), 14 (elbow or triceps extension), and 23 (squat or leg extension)—for dive and push-off strength. In addition to swim strength, water polo players need frog-kick strength—exercise 18 (hip adduction). For throwing strength they should do exercises 2A (standing forward raise), 2D (rotator cuff dumbbell rotation), 2E (rotator cuff pulley exercise), 2F (bent dumbbell pull-back), 14 (triceps extension), and 15 (wrist curls).

Backstrokers should concentrate on exercise 3C (sideways straight-arm pull-down on machine).

Breaststrokers should add exercises 17 (hip abduction) and 18 (hip adduction).

Competitive swimmers who are looking for a combination strength/muscular endurance exercise can try a "reverse pyramid" workout of straight-arm pull-downs on a lat machine. Start with 1 RM, then try a second, then drop the pin to the next weight and do as many reps as possible. Then drop the pin to

> ☑ *Checklist for the Clean and Jerk (an Olympic lift)*
>
> 1. Take a shoulder-width or narrower stance.
> 2. Squat down and grasp the bar slightly wider than shoulder width.
> 3. Keep your back flat at about a 45-degree angle to the floor.
> 4. Keep your shoulders well in front of the bar.
> 5. Lift the bar upward using only your legs (with your back at about the same angle to the floor as in the beginning position).
> 6. Keep the bar close to your shins, and keep your shoulders over the bar. This will keep you in an effective position for the second pull.
> 7. As the bar passes your knees, re-flex your knees.
> 8. Pull the bar upward and move under the bar quickly.
> 9. Begin the jerk motion by flexing your knees and dropping under the bar while pushing it upward.
> 10. Extend your knees and hold until the official declares it a legal lift.

the next lowest weight and repeat to exhaustion. Then drop the pin again until a total of 200 reps have been completed in a short period of time. This is highly efficient but difficult to accomplish. (It takes a lot of "guts" to stick to it, which is why it is called the "gut workout.")

Tennis players should emphasize exercises 2D (rotator cuff dumbbell rotation), 2E (rotator cuff pulley exercise), 2F (bent dumbbell pull-back), 14 (triceps extension), 15 (wrist curls), and 16 (reverse wrist curls).

Track and field offer so many events that each must be addressed separately.

Sprinters, jumpers, and distance runners who need kick strength require extra work on exercises 4D (bent-arm pullover), 7 (hip flexors on high bar or machine), 9 (hip extensors on machine or with a partner), 11 (ankle plantar flexion), and 23 (squat or leg press) or 24 (lunge).

Shot-putters should add exercises 20 (incline bench press at exactly 45 degrees—this is the most important exercise), 15 (wrist curls), 23 (squat or leg press), 24 (lunge), and 28 (power snatch).

Discus throwers should add exercises 2A (forward raise—with the palms facing toward the feet), 2C (bent lateral dumbbell raise), and 17 (hip abduction).

Pole vaulters need strength in nearly every muscle, so they need a lot of extra work, especially exercises 4C (straight-arm pull-down on machine), 5 (all abdominal exercises), 6 (back extension), 7 (hip flexors on high bar or machine), 14 (triceps extension), 21 (overhead barbell press), 22 (pull-down on lat machine), and 28 (power snatch).

Volleyball players should emphasize exercises 2A (standing forward raise), 2D, E, and F (rotator cuff), 11 (ankle plantar flexion), 14 (triceps extension), 15 (wrist curls), and 23 (squat or leg extension), or 24 (lunge).

Checklist for General Muscle Strength

1. Leg strength (squats, calf rises)
2. Shoulder strength (bench press and shoulder press)
3. Upper back (lat exercises)
4. Arm strength (biceps curls and triceps extensions)
5. General body (cleans)
6. Hip (abduction and adduction)
7. Abdominals (curl-ups)
8. Lower back (back extensions)

Weight lifters (Olympic lifts) should work on exercises 15 and 16 (wrist curls), 21 (overhead press), 23 (squat), 25 (upright row), 27 (power clean), and 28 (power snatch). In addition, they should do the clean and jerk, described on page 128, and the snatch (see page 119). Remember, do not attempt to lift maximum weight without knowledgeable supervision

Wrestlers also use nearly every muscle but should emphasize exercises 1 (all neck exercises), 13 (biceps curls), 14 (triceps extension), 15 (wrist curls), 17 hip abduction), 18 (hip adduction), 19 (bench press), 22 (lat pull-downs or chin-ups), 23 (squat or leg extension), and 26 (bent row).

Finally, all athletes who throw overhand (baseball players, quarterbacks, water polo players) should use a high pulley on a machine or an isokinetic machine to approximate the throwing motion.

Cardiovascular Endurance

Most athletes should work on improving cardiovascular endurance, which requires a separate workout. Strength workouts will not provide this type of conditioning.

It is generally agreed that cardiovascular exercise must continue for at least five minutes before benefits begin, with a 20-minute minimum recommended. The exercise should be continuous (such as running, swimming, or cycling) rather than a start-stop activity (such as football, volleyball, or tennis). For athletes, the cardiovascular aspect of the exercise should also include muscular endurance. So while either running or swimming can produce cardiovascular benefits, the swimmer should choose swimming rather than running for a workout, and the runner should choose running. This is because the swimmer needs arm and shoulder muscular endurance while the runner needs leg endurance.

Considerations for the Female Athlete

The difference between male and female bodies is in their potential for developing strength.[1] Male athletes gain strength faster and achieve higher levels of strength than do females. The average woman's absolute body strength is about two-thirds that of the average man's.

One's strength is determined by both quantity and quality of muscle fibers. And while men and women have approximately the same percentage of type I and type IIb (slow-twitch and fast-twitch) muscle fibers, men have larger fibers—especially of the fast-twitch type. This, combined with the larger size of men, gives them more potential for strength.

While the differences of strength are great in the upper body, they are very small for the lower body muscles (hips and legs). This is because women have a greater proportion of their lean body weight below the waist.

Summary

1. An effective posture is aided by correct stretching and strengthening exercises.

2. Every athlete may find it valuable to perform a general body strength workout with exercises for:
   - Shoulders, biceps, and triceps
   - Abdominals, upper back, and lower back
   - Hips and legs

3. Every athlete should develop the specific strength, flexibility, muscular endurance, and cardiovascular endurance necessary to his or her chosen sport. The specific muscular actions that should be emphasized will vary from sport to sport.

---

1 Roundtable, "Strength training and conditioning for the female athlete," *National Strength and Conditioning Association Journal*, 1985, 7(3), 10–29.

10 *Nutrition for Better Conditioning*

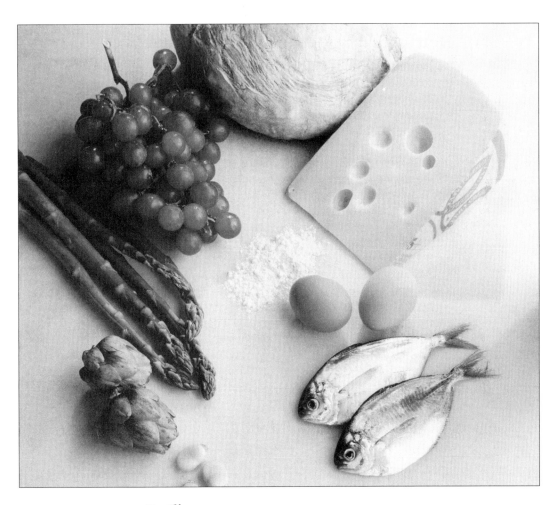

Outline

Nutrition
Protein
Fats
Carbohydrates
Fiber
Vitamins

Checklist for Effective Eating
Minerals
Phytochemicals
Water
Summary

Along and full life requires exercise, an adequate diet, and play—both physical and mental—and a basic understanding of the science of nutrition is essential to healthy living. If you are going to do strength training you will need adequate fuel for your athletic body. This chapter describes the basic elements of good nutrition. In the next chapter we will discuss how to apply these nutritional principles to your diet and weight management.

Nutrition

An informed person is aware of the nutrients necessary for minimal function, and can then put that knowledge into practice by developing a proper diet. Unfortunately, very few people consume even the minimum amounts of each of the necessary nutrients—protein, fat, carbohydrates, vitamins, minerals, and water (the essential nonnutrient). The first three nutrients listed (protein, fat, and carbohydrates) provide the energy required to keep us alive, in addition to making other specific contributions to our bodies.

The calorie measure used in counting food energy is really a kilocalorie— one thousand times larger than the calorie used as a measurement of heat in your chemistry class. In one food calorie (kilocalorie), there is enough energy to heat one kilogram of water one degree Celsius, or to lift 3,000 pounds of weight one foot high. So those little calories you see listed on cookie packages pack a lot of energy.

Most people need about 10 calories per pound of body weight just to stay alive. If you plan to do something other than just lie in bed all day, you probably need about 17 calories per pound of body weight per day in order to keep yourself going. And if you decide to play a couple of hours of singles, you can count on using a whole lot more calories.

For serious bodybuilders or athletes who want to build and keep muscle bulk, there are special requirements for caloric intake. In order to build muscle, you may need to consume 25 to 30 calories per pound of body weight. Then, to maintain the muscle bulk, you can drop to about 20 calories per pound.[1]

The type of calories you take in is also important in muscle building. In the past, bodybuilders and strength athletes often ate large amounts of meat and eggs to get enough protein to make muscle tissue. We now realize that this

Muscle-Maintenance Program of 20 Calories (Kilocalories) per Pound				
Body Weight (Pounds)	Calories per Day	Calories from Carbohydrate (70%)	Calories from Protein (13–16%)	Calories from Fat (12–16%)
140	2800	2000	360–460	340–440
200	4000	2800	510–660	540–690

1 S. M. Kleiner, "Nutrition for muscle builders," *The Physician and Sports Medicine*, August 1997, 25 (8).

Muscle-Building Program of 25 to 30 Calories (Kilocalories) per Pound				
Body Weight (Pounds)	Calories per Day	Calories from Carbohydrate (70%)	Calories from Protein (13–16%)	Calories from Fat (12–16%)
140	3500–4200	2450–2940	455–670	420–672 (90–115 g per day)
200	5000–6000	3500–4200	650–960	600–960 (130–165 g per day)

was a nonsensical approach to muscle building. Only slightly more protein is needed for muscle building—but more carbohydrates are needed. This is because in addition to the protein needed for building the muscles, energy is needed to perform the exercises, and this requires carbohydrates.

Protein

Protein is made up of 22 *amino acids*, which consist of carbon, hydrogen, oxygen, and nitrogen. While both fats and carbohydrates contain the first three elements, nitrogen is found only in protein. Protein is essential for building nearly every part of the body—the brain, heart, organs, skin, muscles, and even the blood.

There are four calories in one gram of protein. Adults require 0.75 grams of protein per kilogram of body weight per day; this translates into one-third a gram of protein per pound. So an easy way to estimate your protein requirements in grams per day would be to divide your body weight by three. For instance, if you weigh 150 pounds, you need about 50 grams of protein per day.

Physically active adults have been thought to require more protein than is recommended by the United States Recommended Daily Allowance (USRDA), which is set at .8 grams per kilogram of body weight per day. In fact, most active people do not need to eat additional protein if 12 to 15 percent of their total calories is protein. Since active individuals need to consume more calories per day than their inactive counterparts due to their increased energy expenditure, active adults who keep their protein intake at around 15 percent of their total calories will eat more protein per day and thereby fulfill their body's protein requirement. Excess protein consumption (above the body's requirement) is broken down and the calories are either burned off or stored as fat.

However, when you are involved in a strenuous strength training regimen, it may be necessary to increase your protein intake percentage, depending on the number of total calories you consume per day. But, as mentioned earlier, the older idea of very large amounts of protein for bodybuilders and strength trainers is no longer accepted.

In order for your body to make any kind of tissue, including muscle, you must first have all of the necessary amino acids. Your body can manufacture some of them, while you must get others from your food. Those amino acids that you must get from your food are called the *essential amino acids*, while the others that you can make are known as the *nonessential amino acids*. During childhood, nine of the 22 amino acids are essential, while in adulthood we acquire the ability to synthesize one additional amino acid, leaving us with eight essential amino acids.

Amino acids cannot be stored in the body, so we need to consume our minimum amounts of protein every day. If adequate protein is not consumed, the body immediately begins to break down tissue (usually beginning with muscle tissue) to release the essential amino acids. If even one essential amino acid is lacking, the other essential ones are not able to work to their capacities. For example, if methionine (the most commonly lacking amino acid) is present at 60 percent of the minimum requirement, the other seven essential amino acids are limited to near 60 percent of their potential. When they are not used, amino acids are excreted in the urine.

Animal products (fish, poultry, and beef) and animal byproducts (milk, eggs, and cheese) are rich in readily usable protein. This means that when you eat animal products or by-products, the protein you consume can be converted into protein in your body because these sources have all of the essential amino acids in them. These foods are called *complete protein sources*.

Incomplete protein sources are any other food sources that provide protein but not all of the essential amino acids. Examples of incomplete proteins include peas and nuts. These food sources must be combined with other food sources that have the missing essential amino acids so that you can make protein in your body. Examples of complementary food combinations are rice and beans or peanut butter on whole wheat bread.

Another reason to be aware of complementary food combinations is that they enhance the absorption of the protein consumed. The person who is aware of the varying qualities of proteins can combine them to take advantage of the strengths of each. For example, if you eat flour at breakfast in the form of a piece of toast or coffee cake and wash it down with coffee, then drank a glass of milk at lunch, each of the protein sources would be absorbed by your body at a lower level. But if you ate bread with the milk at either meal, the higher protein values of both would be absorbed by your body immediately.

Protein supplements are used by some people, particularly weight trainers and athletes. These supplements may not be a good value, however, because they usually fall far short of a good balance of the essential amino acids. Better and cheaper sources of protein if you need a supplement are powdered milk, egg whites (or egg substitutes), milk, or chicken. Any of these may prove less expensive and more nutritious than commercial protein supplements.

Essential Information on Amino Acids

The Essential Amino Acids and Some Foods That Contain Them
- Isoleucine: Fish, beef, organ meats, eggs, shellfish, whole wheat, soya, milk.
- Leucine: Beef, fish, organ meats, eggs, soya, shellfish, whole wheat, milk, liver.
- Lysine: Fish, beef, organ meats, shellfish, eggs, soya, milk, liver.
- Methionine: Fish, beef, shellfish, eggs, milk, liver, whole wheat, cheese.
- Phenylalanine: Beef, fish eggs, whole wheat, shellfish, organ meats, soya, milk.
- Threonine: Fish, beef, organ meats, eggs, shellfish, soya, liver.
- Tryptophan: Soy milk, fish, beef, soy flour, organ meats, shell fish, eggs.
- Valine: Beef, fish, organ meats, eggs, soya, milk, whole wheat, liver.

Amino Acid Requirements[a]

Amino Acid	Mg per Kg per Day	Mg per Pound per Day
Histidine	8–12	3.6–5.4
Isoleucine	10	4.5
Leucine	14	6.4
Lysine	12	5.5
Methionine + cystine[b]	13	6.0
Phenylananine	14	6.4
Threonine	7	3.2
Tryptophan	3.5	1.6
Valine	10	4.5

a Recommended Daily Allowances, 10th ed., Washington, D.C.: National Academy Press, 1989, p. 57.

b Cystine is a nonessential amino acid that can be ingested or can be made from methionine; thus, the two are often listed together.

Fats

Fat is made of carbon, hydrogen, and oxygen. There are nine calories in a gram of fat. In the body, fat is used to develop the myelin sheath that surrounds the nerves. It also aids in the absorption of vitamins A, D, E, and K, which are the fat-soluble vitamins. It serves as a protective layer around our vital organs, and it is a great insulator against the cold. It is also a great concentrated energy source. And of course its most redeeming quality is that it adds flavor and juiciness to food!

Just as protein is broken down into different kinds of nitrogen compounds called amino acids, there are also different kinds of fats. There are three major kinds of fats, or fatty acids: saturated fats, monounsaturated fats, and polyunsaturated fats.

Saturated fats are "saturated" with hydrogen atoms. They are generally solid at room temperature and are most often found in animal fats, eggs, and whole milk products. Since these are the fats that are primarily responsible for raising the blood cholesterol level and hardening the arteries, they should be minimized in your diet.

Monounsaturated fats (oleic fatty acids) have room for two hydrogen ions to double-bond to one carbon. They are liquid at room temperature and are found in great amounts in olive, peanut, and canola (rapeseed) oils. Dietary monounsaturated fats have been shown to help the body excrete dietary cholesterol, thereby contributing a positive effect on atherosclerosis, one type of arteriosclerosis.

Polyunsaturated fats (linoleic fatty acids) have at least two carbon double bonds available, which translates into space for at least four hydrogen ions. Polyunsaturated fats are also liquid at room temperature and are found in the highest proportions in vegetable sources. Safflower, corn, and linseed oils are good sources of this type of fat. Polyunsaturated fatty acids of the omega-3 type may also contribute to the prevention of atherosclerosis.

We eat too much fat. The minimum requirement for fat in the diet is considered to be somewhere between 10 and 20 percent of the total calories consumed. The absolute maximum should be 30 percent, which is the amount now recommended for the American diet. While we as a society are still above this 30 percent value, we have been declining since the 1970s, and we need to keep that trend going. Most of us consume between 35 and 50 percent of our total calories in fats, with a very high percentage in saturated fats—the fats that we want to avoid.

Our high fat intake, most of which is saturated, tends to raise blood cholesterol levels in many people. If you are interested in decreasing the chances of developing hardened arteries by lowering your blood cholesterol level, it is recommended that you follow a diet low in fat (with the saturated fat intake at 10 percent or less of your total diet) and consume less than 300 milligrams of cholesterol daily. Or to put it another way, keep the total calories from fat under a third of your total intake and eat twice as much polyunsaturated and monounsaturated fat as saturated fat.

In the past, companies were allowed to identify the oil in a product on their labels as simply vegetable oil; under the Food and Drug Administration requirements made in 1976, they are now required to note whether it is corn oil, cottonseed oil, soybean oil, and so on, because some oils, even though they are not of animal origin, are very high in saturated fat. Palm kernel oil and coconut oil, often referred to as "tropical oils," are particularly high in saturated fats.

When you buy foods, especially cookies and crackers, always check the type of fat used. Avoid those with palm kernel oil and coconut oil. Also be aware of the hydrogenated oils used. While a hydrogenated safflower or canola oil may still have an acceptable fat ratio, a hydrogenated peanut or cottonseed oil may not contain the desired levels of unsaturated fats. Partially hydrogenated vegetable oils may contribute to the development of heart disease. The dietary use of hydrogenated corn oil stick margarine has been shown to increase LDL cholesterol levels when compared to the use of similar amounts of corn oil, also indicating an increased risk of heart disease.

In terms of controlling one's blood cholesterol level, dietary cholesterol is not as important as saturated fats in your diet. For this reason, saturated fats such as red meats, butter, egg yolks, chicken skin, and other animal fats should be greatly decreased. As an informed consumer, you may want to keep track of both your total fat intake and your intake of saturated fat to become better aware of your potential risk for heart disease. For example, one egg contains 5.6 grams of fat and only 0.7 grams of polyunsaturated fat, while an equal weight of hamburger contains 8.7 grams of fat and only 0.4 grams of polyunsaturated fats.

Carbohydrates

Carbohydrates are made from carbon, hydrogen, and oxygen, just as are fats, but "carbs" are generally a simpler type of molecule. There are four calories in a gram of carbohydrate. If carbohydrates are not utilized immediately for energy as sugar (glucose), they are either stored in the body as glycogen (the stored form of glucose) or synthesized into fat and stored. Some carbohydrates cannot be broken down by the body's digestive processes; these are called fibers and will be discussed later. Digestible carbohydrates, can be separated into two categories: simple and complex. *Simple carbohydrates* are the most readily usable energy source in the body and include such things as sugar, honey, and fruit. These are essential energy sources for your strength training. *Complex carbohydrates* are the starches, which also break down into sugar for energy, but their breakdown is slower than with simple "carbs." Complex carbohydrates also bring with them various vitamins and minerals.

People in the United States often eat too many simple carbohydrates. These are often referred to as "empty calories," because they have no vitamins, minerals, or fibers. While a person who uses a great deal of energy can consume these empty calories without potential weight gain, most of us find these empty calories settling on our hips. The average person consumes 125 pounds of sugar per year, which is equivalent to one teaspoon every 40 minutes, night and day. Since each teaspoon of sugar contains 17 calories, this amounts to 231,000 calories or 66 pounds of potential body fat if this energy is not used as fuel for daily living.

High-carbohydrate diets that are especially high in sugar may be hazardous to one's health. They can increase the amount of triglycerides produced in the liver. These triglycerides are blood fats and are possible developers of hardened arteries. Also, a diet high in simple carbohydrates can lead to obesity, which can then result in the development of late-onset diabetes.

Fiber

Fiber is that part of the foods we take in that is not digestible. Fiber helps to move food through the intestines by increasing their peristaltic action. Vegetable fibers are made up chiefly of cellulose, an indigestible carbohydrate that is the main ingredient in the cell walls of plants. Plant-eating animals, such as cows, can digest cellulose. Meat-eating animals, such as humans, do not have the proper enzymes in their digestive tracts to metabolize cellulose.

Bran—the husks of wheat, oats, rice, rye, and corn—is another type of fiber. Bran is indigestible because of the silica in the outer husks. Some fibers, such as wheat bran, are also insoluble. The major function of fiber is to add bulk to the feces and to speed digested foods through the intestines. This reduces one's risk of constipation, intestinal cancer, appendicitis, and diverticulosis.

Some types of fibers are soluble; that is, they can find and eliminate certain substances such as dietary cholesterol. Pectin, commonly found in raw fruits (especially apple skins), oat and rice brans, and some gums from the seeds and stems of tropical plants (such as guar and xanthin) are examples of soluble fibers that pick up cholesterols as they move through the intestines.

Foods high in fiber are also valuable in weight-reducing diets because when foods pass more quickly through the digestive tract, the time available for absorption is reduced. Fiber also cuts the amount of hunger experienced by a dieter because it fills the stomach. A large salad with a diet dressing might give you very few calories, but it contains enough cellulose to fill your stomach, cut hunger, and move other foods through the intestinal passage.

Food processing often removes natural fiber from our food, and this is one of the primary reasons that we in the western world have relatively low amounts of fiber in our diet. For instance, white bread has only a trace of fiber—about nine grams in a loaf—while old-fashioned whole wheat bread has 70 grams. And when you peel a carrot or an apple, you remove much of the fiber.

Dietitians urge us to include more fiber in our diets. People should be particularly conscious of the benefits of whole-grain cereals, bran, and fibrous vegetables. Root vegetables (carrots, beets, and turnips) and leafy vegetables are very good sources of fiber. The average American diet has between 10 and 20 grams of fiber in it per day. This low level of fiber is believed to account for the fact that we have about twice the rate of colon cancer as do other countries whose citizens eat more fiber. This is why the National Cancer Institute has recommended that we consume between 25 and 35 grams of fiber per day.

Vitamins

Vitamins are organic compounds that are essential in small amounts for the growth and development of animals and humans. They act as enzymes (catalysts) that facilitate many of the body's processes. Although there is controversy about the effects of consuming excess vitamins, nutritionists agree that we need a minimum amount of vitamins for proper functioning.

Checklist for Effective Eating

1. Eat 12 to 15 percent of your diet in proteins, preferably fish, fowl without skin, and beans.
2. Keep your fat intake between 10 and 30 percent of your total calorie intake, with saturated fat intake 10 percent or less and a higher proportion of monounsaturated fat.
3. Most of your diet should be complex carbohydrates (less-refined products) such as whole wheat, fruits, and vegetables.
4. It is recommended that people supplement with antioxidant vitamins (beta carotene, vitamins C and E).

Some vitamins are soluble only in water; others need fat to be absorbed by the body. The water-soluble vitamins, B complex and C, are more fragile than the fat-soluble vitamins, because they are more easily destroyed by the heat of cooking, and if they are boiled, they lose some of their potency into the water. Since they are not stored by the body, they should be included in the daily diet. However, even though they are not stored in the body, it is still possible to ingest too many water-soluble vitamins, leading to kidney stones because of the excess demand placed on the kidneys for processing.

The fat-soluble vitamins, A, D, E, and K, need oils in the intestines to be absorbed by the body. They are more stable than the water-soluble vitamins and are not destroyed by normal cooking methods. Because they are stored in the body, there is the possibility of ingesting too much of them—especially vitamins A and D.

Although nutritional researchers disagree about whether vitamin supplements are necessary, many of them see the necessity for supplementation with the vitamins that neutralize free oxygen radicals. Free oxygen radicals are harmful substances produced by many natural body processes, air pollution, and smoke, and seem to be responsible for some cancers and other diseases. Physical exercise, for all of its benefits, is one producer of free oxygen radicals.

Supplementation with antioxidants (beta carotene, vitamins C and E) reduces free oxygen radicals in the body. Dr. Ken Cooper, the man who coined the term "aerobics" and developed the first world-recognized fitness program, suggests a minimum supplementation of 400 IU of vitamin E, 1,000 mg of vitamin C, and 25,000 of beta carotene daily to counteract the potential damage done to the body by free oxygen radicals.

Minerals

Minerals are usually structural components of the body, but they sometimes participate in certain body processes. The body uses many minerals: phosphorus, calcium, and magnesium for strong teeth and bones; zinc for growth; chromium for carbohydrate metabolism; and copper and iron for hemoglobin production in the blood.

Iron is used primarily in developing hemoglobin, which carries oxygen in red blood cells. Women need more iron (15 milligrams a day) than men until they go through menopause, at which time their iron requirements drop to that of men (12 milligrams a day). Iron deficiency, common in women athletes, may impair athletic performance and should be corrected with supplementation.

Magnesium is the eighth most abundant element on the earth's surface. It seems to help activate enzymes essential to energy transfer. It is crucial for effective contraction of the muscles. Exercise depletes this element, so supplementation may be called for. When it is not present in sufficient amounts, twitching, tremors, and undue anxiety may develop.

Calcium is primarily responsible for building strong bones and teeth. For this reason, it seems obvious that a diet that is chronically low in calcium would have a negative effect on one's bone strength. Low calcium intake results in brittle and porous bones as one gets older, a condition known as osteoporosis. This is diagnosed when bone density shows a loss of 40 percent of the necessary calcium. It happens quite often in older people, especially women who have gone through menopause or have had their ovaries removed, because estrogen seems to protect against bone loss.

In teenage and young adult years, the inclusion of adequate calcium (which may be higher than the current Recommended Daily Allowance, or RDA) can aid in the development of peak bone mass, which can help prevent osteoporosis later on in life. Another contributing factor to osteoporosis is the imbalance of phosphorus to calcium in the typical diet. Calcium and phosphorous work together, and should be consumed on a one-to-one ratio. However, the average diet is much higher in phosphorus than calcium, leading to a leaching of calcium from the bones to make up for this imbalance.

Calcium is also necessary for strong teeth, nerve transmissions, blood clotting, and muscle contractions. Without enough calcium, muscle cramps often result. Skipping milk with its necessary calcium may be the cause of menstrual cramping for some girls. The uterus is a muscle, and muscles need both sodium and calcium for proper contractile functioning.

The major book on nutrition is *Food Values of Portions Commonly Used* by Jean Pennington (Philadelphia: J. B. Lippincott). The 1994 edition was the sixteenth; look for the most recent.

This book lists nearly all foods with their fat, carbohydrate, protein, vitamin, and mineral contents. It also lists foods by amino acid content, vitamin E, and other vitamins and minerals. It is a "must" if you are concerned with evaluating and planning your nutrition.

Phytochemicals

Phytochemicals (phyto is the Greek word for "plant") include thousands of chemical compounds that are found in plants. Some of these are vitamins and many have no known effect on us; however, more and more are being found to be highly beneficial.

In the past, the phytonutrients found in fruits and vegetables were classified as vitamins: Flavonoids were known as vitamin P, cabbage factors (glucosinolates and indoles) were called vitamin U, and ubiquinone was vitamin Q. Tocopherol somehow stayed on the list as vitamin E. The vitamin designation was dropped for other nutrients because specific deficiency symptoms could not be established. "Vita" means "life," so if the compound could not be found to be absolutely essential for life, it was dropped as a "vitamin," but is now classified as a phytochemical.

Various phytochemicals have been found to reduce the chance of cancers developing, reduce the chance of heart attack, reduce blood pressure, and increase immunity factors. Few of these have been reduced to pill form, such as vitamin pills, so they must be consumed in fruits and vegetables daily. It is suggested that each of us consume at least five servings of raw fruits or vegetables daily. Since many of the phytochemicals are heat sensitive, cooking can destroy some or all of the active ingredients.

We are a long way from developing highly effective phytochemical supplements, because there are so many elements and they may be destroyed in the processing. Garlic pills, for example, are available. However, in the deodorized versions, some active ingredients have been removed—they were in the chemicals that give garlic its "aroma."

Several types of phytochemicals are being studied. *Plant sterols* are somewhat similar to the animal sterol cholesterol but are unsaturated. These plant sterols compete for the same sites and thereby lower the blood cholesterol levels by as much as 10 percent. Soy is a good source for such sterols. Most green and yellow vegetables, and particularly their seeds, contain essential sterols.

Phenols have the ability to block specific enzymes that cause inflammation. They also modify the prostaglandin pathways and thereby protect blood platelets from clumping, which reduces the risk of blood clots. Blue, blue-red, and violet colorations seen in berries, grapes, and purple eggplant are due to their phenolic content.

Flavonoids is the name for a large group of compounds found primarily in tea, citrus fruits, onions, soy, and wine. Some can be irritating, but others seem to reduce heart attack risk. For example, the phenolic substances in red wine inhibit oxidation of human LDL cholesterol. The biologic activities of flavonoids include action against allergies, inflammation, free radicals, liver toxins, blood clotting, ulcers, viruses, and tumors.

Terpenes such as those found in green foods, soy products, and grains comprise one of the largest classes of phytonutrients. The most intensely studied terpenes are carotenoids—as evidenced by the many recent studies on beta carotene. Only a few of the carotenoids have the antioxidant properties of beta carotene. These substances are found in bright yellow, orange, and red plant pigments found in vegetables such as tomatoes, parsley, oranges, pink grapefruit, and spinach.

Limonoids are a subclass of terpenes found in citrus fruit peels. They appear to protect lung tissue and aid in detoxifying harmful chemicals in the liver.

Recent research confirms suspicion of the effects of soy products and related foods, which have long been used in Oriental diets. It has long been observed that Oriental women do not experience the problems of menopause, such as hot flashes, that western women commonly endure, but until recently, no theories have been advanced. Now we realize that a major factor is the fact that the Asians eat more vegetables, particularly soybeans.

It is phytoestrogens—plant chemicals that mimic the effects of the female hormone estrogen—that seem to be the major factor. These plant-like estrogens have similar effects to the natural estrogen in reducing heart disease, maintaining brain functions, reducing the incidence of breast cancer, and reducing softening of the bones (osteoporosis). In addition, other positive effects, which may or may not be related to estrogen intake, also occur, such as reduction in cancers (prostate, endometrial, bowel) and the effects of alcohol abuse[2].

Water

Water is called the essential nonnutrient because it has no nutritional value, yet without it we would die. Water makes up approximately 60 percent of the adult body, while an infant's body is nearly 80 percent water. Water cools the body through perspiration, carries nutrients to and waste products from the cells, helps cushion our vital organs, and is an essential element of all body fluids.

The body has about 18 square feet of skin that contains about 2 million sweat glands. On a comfortable day, a person perspires about a half-pint of water. Somebody exercising on a severely hot day may lose as much as seven quarts of water. If this is not replaced, severe dehydration can result. It is therefore generally recommended that we daily drink eight 8-ounce glasses of water or the equivalent in other fluids. This amount is dependent on the climate in which you live, the altitude at which you live, the type of foods that you eat, and the amount of activity that you participate in on a day-to-day basis.

Make sure you go into your workouts well hydrated by drinking 2 cups of fluid two hours before exercise. During exercise, drink 4 to 8 ounces every 15 to 20 minutes. After exercise, replace any further fluid losses with 16 ounces of

---

2 S. A. Bingham et al., "Phyto-oestrogens: Where are we now?" *British Journal of Nutrition*, May 1998, 79(5), 393–406; S. T. Willard and L. S. Frawley, ""Phytoestrogens have agonistic and combinatorial effects on estrogen-responsive gene expression in MCF-7 human breast cancer cells," *Endocrinology*, April 1998, 8(2), 117–121; T. B. Clarkson, "The potential of soybean phytoestrogens for postmenopausal hormone replacement therapy," *Proceedings of the Society of Experimental Biological Medicine*, March 1998, 217(3), 365–368.

fluids. You should also weigh yourself before and after a workout. Any weight loss is fluid and should be replaced as rapidly as possible.

Summary

1. The basic macronutrients are proteins, fats, and carbohydrates.
2. Proteins are made of amino acids. Eight of these are considered to be essential and should be consumed daily.
3. Our bodies need fats, but they should be limited to 10 to 20 percent of our daily calorie intake.
4. Saturated fats and cholesterol are risk factors for heart disease.
5. The greatest percentage of our diets should be in complex carbohydrates, which contain vitamins, minerals, and fiber.
6. While proteins, fats, and carbohydrates (macronutrients) provide most of the nutrients we consume, the micronutrients (vitamins, minerals, and phytochemicals) are also essential.
7. Vitamins break down macronutrients and accomplish other essential body functions.
8. Free oxygen radicals are harmful byproducts of living that can be reduced by some vitamins (beta carotene, vitamins C and E).
9. Minerals are necessary building blocks of the body and are essential in all tissue.
10. Phytochemicals are desirable—and possibly necessary—elements found in plants, and may aid us in obtaining a higher level of nutrition.
11. Vitamin supplementation may be necessary for many people; most of us apparently profit from antioxidant supplementation.
12. Water is essential to all the body's functions; eight glasses of water a day is recommended.

11 *Sensible Eating and Weight Management*

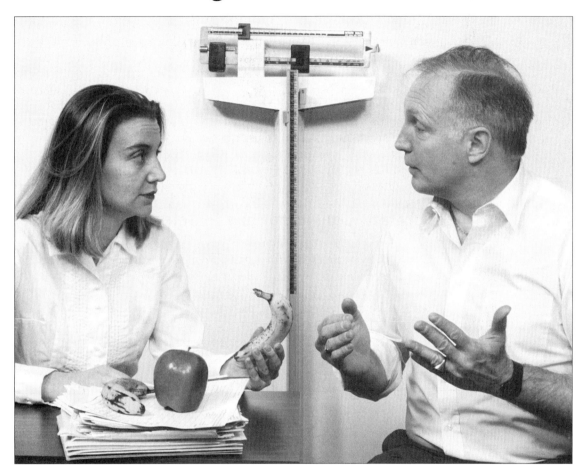

Outline

Important Considerations in
  Selecting Your Diet
Beverages
Food Additives
Vegetarianism
Smart Shopping
Eating and Overeating
How to Lose Weight

*Calories Burned with Various
  Activities*
Eating Disorders
Summary
Self-Test
Bulimia Self-Test
Where to Go for Help
Height and Weight Tables

To eat sensibly, you must understand the basic principles of nutrition discussed in Chapter 10. Necessary nutrients must occur in your diet in proper quantities, and the calories you consume must be the amount necessary in order to maintain your desired weight. If you don't maintain your optimal weight, you may develop obesity and the diseases associated with obesity, such as diabetes, high blood pressure, and heart disease.

There are other factors that the sensible eater must understand. Caloric needs change according to climate and the amount of activity in which the person participates. For example, hot weather necessitates a greater intake of fluids due to the loss of water through perspiration, and you need fewer calories because your body does not need to burn as many calories to maintain its 98.6° Fahrenheit temperature.

A person using a great many calories, such as a serious strength trainer or athlete, needs more carbohydrates, but it is a myth that athletes need a great deal more protein than non-athletes. While caloric needs may nearly double for the athlete who is expending a great deal of energy, protein needs are increased only slightly—usually less than 30 percent.

Important Considerations in Selecting Your Diet

The U.S. Department of Agriculture has devised a suggested diet guide called the Food Guide Pyramid. Its base is grain products, next comes fruits and vegetables, then meats and animal products, and at the top some fats or sweets if needed. There are six food groups in the pyramid:

- Grain products (breads, cereals, pastas): six to eleven servings per day recommended
- Vegetables: three to five servings per day recommended
- Fruits: two to four servings per day recommended
- High-protein meats and meat substitutes (meat, poultry, fish, beans, nuts, tofu/soy, eggs): two to three servings per day recommended
- Milk products: two servings per day for adults, three for children recommended
- Extra calories, if needed, from fats and/or sweets

Grain products provide the carbohydrates needed for quick energy. A serving size is one slice of bread, an ounce of dry cereal, or a half-cup of cooked cereal, pasta, or rice. Daily needs are six to eleven servings.

Grains are rich in B vitamins, some minerals, and fiber. Whole grains are the best sources of fibers. Refining grains or polishing rice reduces the fiber, the mineral content, and the B vitamins. This occurs in white and wheat bread (not whole wheat), pastas, pastries, and white rice. Flour is often refortified with three of the B complex vitamins, but seldom with the other essential nutrients.

If you want to reduce your cholesterol level, thereby reducing your chances of heart disease, reduce your chances of developing gallstones, or have a softer bowel movement, eat more of the soluble fibers (oat bran cereals, whole grain

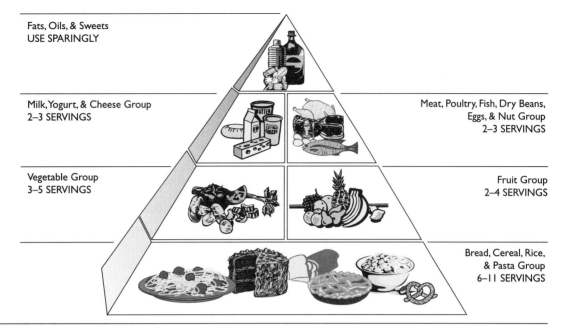

The Food Guide Pyramid

bread with oats, rice bran, carrots, potatoes, apples, and citrus juices that contain pulp). If your concern is reducing your risk of intestinal cancers, appendicitis, and diverticulosis, eat more of the insoluble fibers (whole wheat breads and cereals, corn cereals, prunes, beans, peas, nuts, most vegetables, and polished rice).

Vegetables are rich in fibers, beta carotene, some vitamins, and minerals. Among the most nutritious vegetables are broccoli, carrots, peas, peppers, and sweet potatoes. If you are trying to lose weight, many vegetables are high in water and in fibers but low in calories. Among these are all greens (lettuce, cabbage, celery) as well as cauliflower. Actually, most vegetables are quite low in calories. You need three to five servings daily; a serving size is a half-cup of raw or cooked vegetables or a cup of raw leafy vegetables.

Fruits are generally high in vitamin C and fiber, and they are also relatively low in calories. You should have two to four servings daily; a serving size is one-fourth cup of dried fruit, a half-cup of cooked fruit, three-quarters cup of fruit juice, a whole piece of fruit, or a wedge of a melon.

Protein sources such as meats, egg whites, nuts, and beans are also high in minerals and vitamins B-6 and B-12. You need two to three servings a day; a serving is two and one-half ounces of cooked meat, poultry or fish, two egg whites, four tablespoons of peanut butter, one and one-fourth cups of cooked beans. A McDonald's "Quarter-Pounder" would give you two servings. The hidden eggs in cakes and cookies also count. The best meat products to eat are fish, egg whites, and poultry without the skin.

Red meat not only has a relatively low quality of protein (ranked after egg white, milk, fish, poultry, and organ meats), but it is linked to both cancers (two and a half times the risk for colon cancer) and heart disease. It also carries a great amount of fat, even if the fat on the outside is trimmed off. There is also a lot of cholesterol in the meat and fat of all land animals. Taking the skin off poultry greatly reduces the amount of fat and cholesterol that will be consumed, because poultry carry much of their fat next to the skin.

Of the animal proteins, fish has a higher quality of protein than meat or poultry. Also, fish are able to convert polyunsaturated linolenic fatty acids from plants they eat into omega 3 oils, which work to prevent heart disease by reducing cholesterol and by making the blood less likely to clot in the arteries. They do this by interfering with the body's production of the prostaglandin thromboxane, which increases blood clotting.

Milk and milk products (cheeses, yogurt, ice cream) are high in calcium and protein as well as in some minerals (potassium and zinc) and riboflavin. Adults need two servings daily, while children need three; a serving is one cup of milk or yogurt, one and one-half ounces of cheese, two cups of cottage cheese, one and one-half cups of ice cream, or one cup of pudding or custard.

Fats and sweets are positioned at the top of the pyramid of foods. They should be eaten only if a person needs extra calories. Consuming more fat than the recommended maximum of 30 percent of one's diet can be quite harmful—particularly in causing cancers and hardened arteries. Most researchers suggest a maximum of 10 to 20 percent of the diet in fats, with most in the form of monounsaturated and polyunsaturated fatty acids.

Sweets may assist in the development of tooth caries (cavities), but are not otherwise harmful if calories are not a problem for you. An athlete consuming 5,000 calories in a day can probably eat candy bars and ice cream, but the person attempting to control their weight should avoid them.

In addition to merely consuming the right proportions of foods, a concerned person would implement several other precautions:

- Avoid milk fat by drinking nonfat milk and milk products; eating ice milk (3 percent fat) or frozen desserts made without milk fat; and eating no-fat or low-fat cheeses. Half of the calories in whole milk come from the 3 ½ percent of the milk that is fat. Low-fat milk is reduced in fat calories by 40 percent. When low-fat milk is advertised as 98 percent fat-free, it is not that much better than whole milk, which is 96 ½ percent fat-free. The fats in milk are highly saturated—the worst kind of fat—yet the protein quality of milk is second only to egg whites.
- Avoid egg yolks because they contain a great deal of cholesterol and saturated fat. They are second only to caviar (fish eggs) in cholesterol content. Egg whites, on the other hand, have the highest rating for protein quality and are one of the best things you can eat.
- Reduce salt, because it is related to high blood pressure; and sugars, because they give "empty" calories—calories without other nutrients such as vitamins or fiber.

- Reduce fats to between 10 and 20 percent of your total calories. Normal salad dressings contain about 70 calories per tablespoon. If calories are a problem, use fat-free dressing or vinegar or lemon juice only. Rather than a butter or margarine, buy a good tasty whole-grain bread and eat it without grease. If you must use grease, use olive oil, or perhaps olive oil and balsamic vinegar as they serve in many Italian restaurants. If calories are not a concern and you like sweets, use jelly or jam.

- Never fry foods in oil; use a non-stick pan. If you must have an oil, use canola (rapeseed), olive, or safflower oil. Stay away from all fried foods, including potato chips. Fried foods not only add calories and saturated fats, but they also increase one's chances for intestinal cancers—as do all fats.

Beverages

Beverages make up a large part of our diet. We often don't think too much about the kinds of liquids we drink. The most nutritious drinks have been rated by the Center for Science in the Public Interest according to the amount of fat and sugar (higher content = lower rating), and their amount of protein, vitamins, and minerals (higher content = higher rating). Here are some sample results: skim or nonfat milk was rated +47, whole milk +38 (the lower rating was because of its fat content), orange juice +33, Hi-C +4, coffee 0, coffee with cream –1, coffee with sugar –12, Kool-Aid –55, and soft drinks –92.

Milk is the best beverage for most people. Children should have three to four cups each day, while adults should drink two cups. Our need for milk can be satisfied by other dairy products. For example, two cups of milk are equivalent to three cups of cottage cheese or five large scoops of ice cream. (Of course, this choice may *taste* the best, but there are obvious drawbacks to eating five scoops of ice cream every day!) In addition to its nutritional value as a developer of bones and organs, milk has been found to help people sleep. People who drink milk at night go to sleep more quickly, and sleep longer and sounder. This is because of the high content of the amino acid tryptophan, which makes serotonin, the neurotransmitter (brain chemical) associated with relaxation and calming.

Coffee contains several ingredients that may be harmful to the body. There are stimulants such as caffeine and the xanthines, as well as oils that seem to stimulate the secretion of excess acid in the stomach. And there are diuretics that eliminate water and some nutrients, such as calcium, from the body. Even two cups a day increases the risk of bone fractures[1]. A factor that may add to the risk of bone fractures is that people who drink more coffee usually drink little or no milk.

---

1 E. Barrett-Connor, "Caffeine and bone fractures," *Journal of the American Medical Association*, January 26, 1994.

Caffeine is found in coffee, tea, and cola and many other drinks. Brewed coffee contains 100 to 150 milligrams of caffeine per cup (mg/cup), instant coffee about 90 mg/cup, tea between 45 and 75 mg/cup, and cola drinks from 40 to 60 mg/cup. Decaffeinated coffee is virtually free of caffeine, containing only two to four mg/cup. The therapeutic dose of caffeine given to people who have overdosed on barbiturates is 43 milligrams. Yet a cup of coffee contains up to 150 milligrams of caffeine!

Caffeine is a central nervous system stimulant. It elevates your blood pressure and constricts your blood vessels, both of which effects may assist in the development of high blood pressure. It has also been reported that excess caffeine in coffee, tea, and cola drinks can produce the same symptoms found in someone suffering from psychological anxiety, including nervousness, irritability, occasional muscle twitching, sensory disturbances, diarrhea, insomnia, irregular heartbeat, a drop in blood pressure, and occasionally failures of the blood circulation system.

Coffee is an irritant. The oils in coffee irritate the lining of the stomach and the upper intestines. People who drink two or more cups of coffee per day increase their chances of getting ulcers by 72 percent over non–coffee drinkers. Decaffeinated coffee is no more soothing to the ulcer patient than the regular blend, because both types increase the acid secretions in the stomach. Since an ulcer patient's acid secretion is not as high when caffeine alone is ingested (when compared to the acid levels after the ingestion of decaffeinated coffee), some other ingredient in coffee is thought to be responsible for these increased stomach acid levels.

Tea is not as irritating as coffee, but it does contain some caffeine and tannic acid, which can irritate the stomach. If you drink large amounts of tea, you should either take it with milk to neutralize the acid or add ice to dilute it. Green tea, the type commonly drunk in Asia, contains polyphenols, which appear to be antioxidants and may reduce cancer incidence. Black tea, the kind commonly drunk in Europe and America, has less of these protective substances[2]. Not much is known about the effects of herbal teas.

Alcohol contains seven calories per gram. These calories contain no nutritional elements, but they do contribute to your total caloric intake. Since alcoholic drinks are surprisingly high in calories, they contribute to the overweight problems of many individuals. People who drink alcoholic beverages and eat a balanced diet will probably consume too many calories. If they drink but cut down on eating, they may not develop a weight problem, but they will probably develop nutritional deficiencies that can result in severe illness. Alcohol is also a central nervous system depressant, which causes a decrease in one's metabolism.

2 *University of California, Berkeley Wellness Letter*, January 1992, pp. 1–2.

In addition to the normal dangers of alcohol in creating alcoholism and destroying brain cells, there are other considerations in drinking. Beer or ale, because of their carbonation, have the effect of neutralizing stomach acid. This can increase the acids secreted by the stomach, causing ulcers.

Food Additives

Sugar is a negative for most people. In fact it is probably the most harmful additive to the foods that we in the United States eat. We average about 125 pounds of sugar per person per year. This gives us a lot of excess calories that, if not used for energy, will be stored as fat. As discussed previously, if we exceed our desired weight and become obese, we will have increased health risks.

Salt can be a dangerous food additive, yet most people do not consider adding salt to their food to be a health risk. But when you look at populations as a whole, it seems obvious that the higher the salt intake, the greater the frequency of high blood pressure.

Many manufacturers add salt to enhance the taste of food, and sodium is often high in processed or canned foods. While the desired intake is between one and two grams (1,000 and 2,000 milligrams), the average daily intake in America is five grams. The potential negative effect of a high sodium intake can be combated by ingesting a high level of potassium. However, the desired recommended daily allowance for potassium, 2.5 grams, is not met by the average American, who consumes only 0.8 to 1.5 grams daily. Most of our foods follow this same pattern—too high in sodium and too low in potassium.

Preservatives added to foods lengthen storage life and prevent disease-causing germs from multiplying. Most are harmless, and some give protection against intestinal cancers. Some, however, such as the nitrates in hot dogs, have been implicated in causing cancer. Nevertheless, the disease of botulism, which they prevent, is far more of a danger than that posed by the nitrates.

Vitamins and minerals have been added to food for years. In 1973, the Food and Drug Administration suggested that more iron be added to enrich flour after they found that iron is often low in our diets. Vitamins A and D are added to skim milk to make it nonfat milk—milk that has all of the nutrients of whole milk but without the fat. Vitamins A and D are fat soluble and stay in the fat when it is removed to make skim milk.

Vegetarianism

When vegetarians are careful about their dietary intakes, they may prove to be healthier than nonvegetarians. One study comparing healthy vegetarians to nonvegetarians found that healthy vegetarians had lower blood sugar and cholesterol levels than did their closely matched nonvegetarian counterparts.

Smart Shopping

Shopping for low-fat foods requires a sharp eye. If you are looking for a low-fat food, look at the total grams of fat, multiply by nine (nine calories per gram of fat), then divide that by the total number of calories in the food. (For example, if a food has three grams of fat, nine times that equals 27 total calories from fat. If the food has a total of 270 calories, then the percentage of fat calories is 10 percent.) If the food has one of the new food labels, it will list both the number of fat values and the approximate percentage of fat calories per serving. You want to keep your daily total percentage of fat below 30 percent to decrease your risk of developing heart disease. Even better than the suggested maximum of 30 percent is keeping the total to 10 or 20 percent fat.

Many foods, particularly low-fat liquids such as salad dressings without oil, have replaced the oil with some gums. Guar, locust bean, and xanthine gums are soluble fibers that help remove cholesterol from the intestines. So you get a double advantage—no fat and some cholesterol-removal substances.

The food label lists ingredients according to their content in the product. The higher on the list of ingredients, the more of that item is present in the food. So if the product lists wheat flour first, there is no problem. But if it lists eggs or hydrogenated oils second, the food may be too high in fat. And if you are watching your sodium intake, remember to look for salt on the list.

Eating and Overeating

People eat to nourish their bodies. But in America many people eat to reduce stress. We may not be satisfied in our work, at school, or in our relationships, but we can be satiated with food. Filling our stomachs can make us feel that in at least one part of our lives we are totally satisfied. When we eat to relieve stress, we will probably take in more calories than we need for living—but even worse, stress eating often means junk foods. It is much more intelligent to exercise to relieve stress.

Gaining weight is a desire for some people. The focus of weight gain should be on increasing lean body weight, that is, increasing muscle mass, not fat. To gain weight in muscle, the best method is to do resistance-type exercise, such as strength training. In addition, you must ensure that you eat enough protein in order to give your body the building blocks it needs to make more muscle (although it is not necessary to eat excessive protein).

Being overweight is a more common concern than is being underweight. While some people are overweight, some are obese. For example, 35 percent of women are 20 percent overweight.[3] Of people who are obese, one in 20 has a genetic factor or a problem in physical malfunctioning, such as an underactive thyroid, a problem with the hypothalamus, or one of the other centers of the brain that deals with whether or not we feel full or hungry. There are medical procedures

---

3 *Harvard Women's Health Watch*, November 1994, p. 4.

that can help these people. In cases where the metabolism is slowed, such as by an underactive thyroid gland, doctors can administer the proper hormone to increase metabolism back into what is considered a normal range.

Another cause of obesity is thought to be the number of fat cells in a person's body. This is known as the *set point theory*. It is thought that the more fat cells one has, the more one is driven to eat to maintain these fat cells. The number of fat cells one has is generally set after puberty.

For others, obesity is caused by overeating to an extreme degree. However, according to the Harvard University Nutrition Department, most people are overfat because they don't exercise, not because they overeat. Overeating coupled with a lack of exercise is a sure way to become obese.

Since it is the amount of body fat that a person carries that is the true culprit of disease, it is preferable to refer to this health risk as being overfat rather than being overweight. Many bodybuilders may be overweight when compared to the height/weight charts commonly used to measure health risks by insurance companies, but they are not overfat.

Determining if you are overfat can be done in several ways. The most common method is to look at yourself in a mirror. If you look fat, you may be fat. Another way is to pinch the fat you carry just below the skin. If you can pinch an inch, you are probably carrying too much fat. Professionals often use skin calipers to measure the amount of fat people carry in four to seven designated spots on the body, or they use underwater weighing or bioelectrical impedence.

Once your body fat percentage is determined, you can then find out what a healthy weight would be for you. Men are usually considered healthy if their body fat is in the range of 10 to 15 percent, while women are healthy if they fall between 18 to 25 percent body fat. Men are considered overfat if their body fat is over 20 percent, while women are overfat if their body fat is over 30 percent. Women require more fat than men do because of their menstrual cycle. If a woman falls below 12 percent body fat, she may become amenorrheic (lose her regular menstrual cycle).

Should You Lose Weight?

Before you decide to lose weight, you first need to determine whether your are overweight due to being overfat. From a health point of view, it is your proportion of fat and lean body mass that is most important.

How to Lose Weight

The wisest approach to losing weight would be to find out why you are overweight. If it is genetic, perhaps medical help is needed. If you eat because of stress, you should find another way to relieve stress, such as exercise or relaxation techniques or, if you must have something in your mouth, try gum or a low-calorie food. If your problem is a lack of exercise, start an effective exercise program. If you consume too many calories, you will need to change your diet.

Don't even start a weight-loss program if you are not willing to make lifestyle changes for the rest of your life. The great majority of dieters refuse to make such a commitment. That is why 40 percent of women and 25 percent of men are on a diet at any one time and the average American goes on 2.3 diets a year, and it is also why 95 percent of dieters regain all of their lost weight within five years. The average diet is just not successful.

In all likelihood, if you adopt the habits of effective exercise and a low-fat and low-alcohol eating pattern, the pounds will drop off. Losing weight just for the sake of being thinner seldom works for very long. You have to determine whether you honestly want a healthier lifestyle or just to look better for the summer. A pattern of continually gaining and losing weight is frustrating and probably not worth the effort. But a true lifestyle change to healthy eating and regular exercise will pay many mental, physical, and social dividends.

We must recognize that the fat we wear comes primarily from the fat we eat. Because carbohydrates are so efficiently converted to sugar glucose, they are used first for energy in the body. To convert carbohydrates to fat, about 23 percent of the energy is used to make the conversion. Protein, if not used, will normally be converted into sugars and will be the second source of available energy. But the fat you eat uses only 3 percent of its food value in the conversion to body fat.

So 25 grams of carbohydrate, which will yield 100 calories (at 4 calories a gram), is reduced by 23 percent of the calories used to convert them to body fat. But fats consumed in your food are different. Eleven grams of fat (at nine calories per gram) is 99 calories, but it only takes 3 percent of those calories to convert it all to body fat, and 96 calories of body fat can be deposited. So 100 calories of carbohydrates, if not used for energy, will become about 8.5 grams of body fat, but 100 calories of fat from the diet will become about 10.75 grams of body fat.

To lose one pound of fat per week, you must have a net deficit of 500 calories per day; one pound of fat contains 3,500 calories. You may choose to achieve this solely by decreasing your food intake by 500 calories per day.

You could also choose to increase your activity level to burn off 500 calories a day. Keep in mind that it takes a great deal of energy to achieve this goal, and it can be dangerous for you to embark on such a strenuous exercise program if you are not currently exercising. It is best to combine calorie reduction with exercise to achieve your goal. Aerobic exercise will keep your metabolism up as you lose the fat, and you won't have to restrict your calories as much because you will be burning off energy each time you exercise.

Playing singles tennis burns about 3.4 calories per pound per hour. For a 150-pound person, this is about 510 calories per hour.

We now know that calories are used both during and after exercise. The longer and more vigorous the exercise, the longer one's metabolism is increased, so that for more hours after the exercise is completed, the calorie expenditure will be increased over normal. While this increase in calories burned after one has finished exercising is not a large amount, it is still an increase over one's resting metabolism, and a calorie burned is a calorie burned!

✓ Calories Burned with Various Activities

	Calories per pound per hour	Calories expended by 150 lb. person in 20 minutes
Sleeping	0.36	18.0
Sitting at rest	0.55	27.5
Sitting at work	0.60	30.0
Light exercise (housework)	1.00	50.0
Walking	1.20	60.0
Jogging (slow)	1.75	87.5
Volleyball (recreational 6-person)	1.50	75.0
Tennis	3.40	170
Weight training	3.09	154

Some people think that exercising will make them eat more. A quarter-mile to a mile of jogging or a good set of tennis games will have no measurable effect on the total intake of calories. In fact, by exercising just before a meal, you can dull your appetite and decrease your desire for more calories.

Eating Disorders

Anorexia nervosa is starvation by choice. This is a disease primarily seen in young women. It afflicts nearly one in a hundred women, although 5 to 10 percent of its victims are male. In this disease, the person goes on a diet and refuses to stop, no matter how thin he or she gets. About one out of ten people who have this disorder end up starving themselves to death. The disease has a psychological basis, but its physical effects are very real. Medical care, usually hospitalization, is generally required.

After the anorexic begins the severe dieting routine, symptoms of starvation may set in, leading to a number of physical problems. Abnormal thyroid, adrenal, and growth hormone functions are not uncommon. The heart muscle becomes weakened. Amenorrhea occurs in women and girls due to the low percentage of body fat. Blood pressure may drop. Anemia is common due to the lack of protein and iron ingested. The peristalsis of the intestines may slow and the lining of the intestines may atrophy. The pancreas often becomes unable to secrete many of its enzymes. Body temperature may drop. The skin may become dry and there can be an increase of body hair in the body's attempt to keep itself warm. And for 10 percent of sufferers, the result is death.

Because dieting is such a common occurrence in our society, anorexia is often difficult to diagnose until the person has entered the advanced stages of the disease. However, other symptoms such as moodiness, being withdrawn, obsessing about food but never being seen eating it, and constant food preparation may be observed by those close to the anorexic. Once diagnosed, there are a number of medical and psychological therapies that can be effective.

Bulimia, or *bulimia nervosa*, is more common than anorexia. The person with bulimia restricts calorie intake during the day, but binges on high-fat, high-calorie foods at least twice a week. Following the binge, the person purges in an attempt to get rid of the excess calories just consumed. Purging techniques include vomiting, laxatives, fasting, and excessive exercise. Some experts do not consider the behavior bulimic until it has persisted for about three months with two or more binges per week during that time. Estimates based on various surveys of college students and others indicate that between 5 and 20 percent of women may be bulimic. It is also more common among men than is anorexia.

Bulimia, like anorexia, stems from a psychological problem. However, in some cases there may also be a link to physical abnormalities. The neurotransmitters serotonin and norepinephrine seem to be involved, as does the hormone cholecystokinin, which is secreted by the hypothalamus and makes a person feel that enough food has been eaten.

Physical symptoms to look for depend on the type of purging technique used. The bulimic who induces vomiting can have scars on the back of the knuckles, mouth sores, gingivitis, tooth decay, a swollen esophagus, and chronic bad breath. The bulimic who uses laxatives has constant diarrhea, which can cause irreparable damage to the intestines. All bulimics run the risk of throwing off their electrolytes (minerals involved in muscle contractions) as a result of constant dehydration. It is this imbalance of electrolytes that can cause the bulimic to have abnormal heart rhythms and that can induce a heart attack.

Female athletes sometimes develop problems called the "female athletic triad,"[4] or a combination of eating disorders, osteoporosis, and amenorrhea. It is caused by the hard training practiced by competitive athletes or dancers and the desire to keep weight low, which often results in inadequate nutrition. Weight loss is sometimes achieved by bulimic methods. The result is weight that is too low, a loss of calcium from the bones, and a lack of healthy menstruation.

These problems are most likely to occur in activities in which low weight is an advantage, such as dancing, distance running, figure skating, and gymnastics, and it is more prevalent among athletes in individual sports than in team sports. Males, with the exception of competitive wrestlers, do not often experience the need to eat less.

Muscle dysmorphia is a newly described condition in which male and female bodybuilders see themselves as underdeveloped no matter how muscular they actually are. Several studies have indicated that this is more common than might be assumed. When it occurs, it can cause psychological distress that can

4 Aurelia Nattiv, Barbara Drinkwater, et al. "The female athletic triad," *Clinics in Sports Medicine: The Athletic Woman*, W. B. Saunders: Philadelphia, 13(2), April 1994, 405–418.

affect their lives, both in their social and their occupational functioning. It may lead to an abnormal desire for excess workouts and to steroid usage.[5]

Summary

1. Sensible eating requires some understanding of the science of nutrition.
2. Following the guidelines of the Food Pyramid will generally give a person an adequate diet.
3. Skim or nonfat milk is the best beverage.
4. Salt and sugar are the most common food additives.
5. Many people overeat and become overfat.
6. Most overfat people can lose weight through an effective diet and adequate exercise.
7. Eating disorders seem to be prevalent; anorexia nervosa and bulimia are the major eating disorders.

Self-Test

Write in the number that best describes your eating habits:

3—Almost always   2—Sometimes   1—Almost never

____ 1. Do you eat three or more pieces of fruit per day? (Fruit juice counts as one piece.)
____ 2. Do you eat a minimum of three servings of vegetables each day—including a green leafy or orange vegetable?
____ 3. Do you eat three or four milk products (such as milk, cheese, yogurt) per day?
____ 4. Do you eat a minimum of six servings of grain products (breads, cereal, pasta) each day?
____ 5. Do you eat breakfast?
____ 6. Do you eat fish at least three times per week?
____ 7. Do you avoid fried foods, including potato chips and french fries?
____ 8. Do you eat fast food fewer than three times per week?
____ 9. Are the milk products you consume made from nonfat milk?
____ 10. Do you avoid high-sugar foods and highly refined carbohydrates such as sweet rolls, cookies, nondiet sodas, candy, etc.?

Your Score

25–30   You are balancing your diet well.
18–24   Your diet needs to be improved.
10–17   Your diet is unhealthy.

---

5 H. G. Pope, et al., "Muscle dysmorphia: An unrecognized form of body dysmorphia disorder," *Psychosomatics*, Nov.–Dec., 1997, 38(6), 548–557.

Bulimia Self-Test

Write "Never," "Sometimes," or "Often" to describe your weight-control practices:

____ 1. Is your life a series of constant diets?

____ 2. Do you vomit or take laxatives or diuretics to control your weight?

____ 3. Do you alternate periods of eating binges with fasts to control your weight?

____ 4. Does your weight fluctuate by as much as 10 pounds because of eating habits?

____ 5. Have you ever had a "food binge" during which you ate a large amount of food in a short period of time?

____ 6. If you "binged," was it on high-calorie food such as ice cream, cookies, donuts, or cake?

____ 7. Have you ever stopped a binge by vomiting, sleeping, or experiencing pain?

____ 8. Do you think your eating habits vary from the average person's?

____ 9. Are you out of control with your eating habits?

____10. Are you close to 100 pounds overweight because of your eating habits?

If you marked two or more of the above questions "Often," you may have a serious eating disorder called *bulimia*.

Where to Go for Help

Anorexia Bulimia Treatment Education Center: 800-33-ABTEC

Bulimia Anorexia Self-Help: 800-227-4785

Low-fat diet gourmet meals are possible. Send for the free *Metropolitan Cookbook.* Write to: Health and Welfare Department, Metropolitan Life Insurance Co., 1 Madison Avenue, New York, NY 10010) . Or buy the American Heart Association's cookbook.

Height and Weight Table: Men*

Height	Small Frame	Medium Frame	Large Frame
5'2"	128–134	131–141	138–150
5'3"	130–136	133–143	140–153
5'4"	132–138	135–145	142–156
5'5"	134–140	137–148	144–160
5'6"	136–142	139–151	146–164
5'7"	138–145	142–154	149–168
5'8"	140–148	145–157	152–172
5'9"	142–151	148–160	155–176
5'10"	144–154	151–163	158–180
5'11"	146–157	154–166	161–184
6'0"	149–160	157–170	164–188
6'1"	152–164	160–174	168–192
6'2"	155–168	164–178	172–197
6'3"	158–172	167–182	176–202
6'4"	162–176	171–187	181–207

*Weights at ages 25 to 59 based on lowest mortality. Weight in pounds according to frame (in indoor clothing weighing 5 lbs.; shoes with 1" heels).
Source: 1999 Metropolitan Life Insurance Company height and weight tables.

Height and Weight Table: Women†

Height	Small Frame	Medium Frame	Large Frame
4'10"	102–111	109–121	118–131
4'11"	103–113	111–123	120–134
5'0"	104–115	113–126	122–137
5'1"	106–118	115–129	125–140
5'2"	108–121	118–132	128–143
5'3"	111–124	121–135	131–147
5'4"	114–127	124–138	134–151
5'5"	117–130	127–141	137–155
5'6"	120–133	130–144	140–159
5'7"	123–136	133–147	143–163
5'8"	126–139	136–150	146–167
5'9"	129–142	139–153	149–170
5'10"	132–145	142–156	152–173
5'11"	135–148	145–159	155–176
6'0"	138–151	148–162	158–179

†Weights at ages 25 to 59 based on lowest mortality. Weight in pounds according to frame (in indoor clothing weighing 3 lbs.; shoes with 1" heels).
Source: 1999 Metropolitan Life Insurance Company height and weight tables.

12 *Ergogenics*

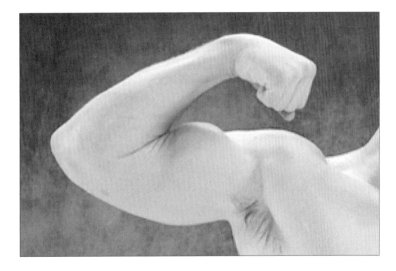

Outline

Aids to Building Muscle
Possible Steroid Side Effects
Increasing Anaerobic Capacity
Fluid and Carbohydrate Replacement
International Olympic Committee Medical Code
Muscle Recovery and Pain Reduction
Endurance Enhancement
Summary

Ergogenic means "work enhancing" or "energy producing." So ergogenic aids are whatever facilitate progress toward strength, bulk development, or aerobic or anaerobic work. They can range from legal vitamin pills to illegal steroids.

Supplementation of legal substances can help to improve performance, to avoid fatigue, or to live longer. This supplementation is generally specific. One supplement may work on the fast-twitch (type IIb) muscle fibers, which are used in weight lifting and sprinting. Another may work on the slow-twitch (type I) fibers, which are used in endurance activities such as long-distance running, dancing, or soccer. Still another supplement may provide the necessary building blocks for bones and other tissues. On the other hand, certain ergogenic aids, such as steroids, can affect an athlete's chance of injury by increasing the risk.

Aids to Building Muscle

Building muscle is done by making certain that the diet has sufficient amounts of high-quality protein. This is best accomplished through high-protein foods. Protein pills are a waste of money; egg whites, nonfat or powdered milk, fish, and chicken contain more and better protein for less money. Certain vitamins and minerals are also essential in building muscle tissue (see Chapter 10). (Of course, if you want to build muscle, you must also work with resistance exercises effectively.)

Nutrition Supplements

Extra meals can add more protein, carbohydrates, vitamins, and minerals to one's diet. An extra meal can range from the eggs, bananas, and milk consumed by the main character in the "Rocky" films, to commercially made, high-protein "diet" drinks, to liquid meals specifically made for athletes and weight trainers.

Tthe commercially available meals may be made from soy protein or from milk products. For those people with a milk allergy, the soy products are preferable. However, for those who can drink milk, the milk protein is a much higher quality than the soy protein because of its amino acid ratio.

Amino acids are often used as supplements to make certain that there is sufficient protein in the body to develop the desired muscle bulk. The advantage of amino acid supplements over high-protein meals is that such meals generally include a great deal of fat, while the amino acids are fat-free. A cheaper and better source of high protein, however, is dry nonfat milk powder or low-fat cottage cheese.

High-carbohydrate foods can be taken before or after a workout to replace the glycogen stores in the muscles. Those products with simpler glucose molecules seem more effective in replacing muscle glycogen than the products that use sugar as the carbohydrate source.

Vitamin and mineral supplements are often used by weight trainers to make certain that they are getting enough of the necessary vitamins and minerals. The one-a-day, time-release type is best. However, most athletes probably get enough vitamins and minerals in their basic diets—with the exception of the antioxidants and, for women, iron. Women's need for iron is nearly double that of men.

Supplementing with the antioxidents is recommended. Since free oxygen radicals are produced continually by the body, and their production is increased by exercise, it is wise to take additional vitamin C, E, and beta carotene.

Steroids

The use of *androgenic steroids*—steroids that are similar to testosterone or the human growth hormone—to build muscle is not recommended for the average person or the athlete. These steroids are legitimately given to people who have a medical need for more testosterone or the growth hormone, because they do not secrete enough of the hormones naturally. But their illicit use has gone on for many years among bodybuilders and athletes for whom strength is a major concern. These people generally take a much higher dosage than those who have a medical need for the hormones.

When steroids are taken, the hypothalamus, the part of the brain that monitors and controls many body functions, picks up the signal that there are too many male hormones in the body. It may then signal the pituitary gland, the adrenals, and the testicles to stop producing their hormones. When the steroid user stops using the drug, the body may have difficulty adjusting to making its own hormones again.

The various steroids may indeed stimulate muscle growth, but they can have negative side effects, which vary from drug to drug. (See the box "Possible Steroid Side Effects" on the next page.) These effects may be somewhat mild, such as headaches, dizziness, or nosebleeds; or they may be very serious, ranging from bone brittleness to liver and kidney damage. Men and women may experience alterations in their reproductive organs or functions, and many people who use the drugs note an increase in their aggressiveness. Teenage boys who take steroids to develop bodies that they think are more attractive to girls may develop early hardening of their bones and, consequently, stunting of growth.

Obviously, the negative effects of steroids far outweigh any benefits. That is why their use, except by prescription, is against the law. Nevertheless, most steroids are obtained illegally. To compound the problem, some bodybuilders take 10 to 20 times the amount that would give them maximum results. They have mistakenly assumed that more is better, when in fact an excess sometimes slows growth and strength development.

While there is no question that steroids add muscle bulk, studies indicate that there is very little difference between how much more one can gain with steroids than with good food. So anyone interested in strength and bulk gain

---

Possible Steroid Side Effects

For the liver: Cancer, jaundice, tumors, pelosis hepatitis.

For the cardiovascular system: High blood pressure, changes in cholesterol levels, heart disease, anaphylactic shock, septic shock, death.

For the reproductive system: Atrophy of the genital organs, possible swelling of the genitals, sexual dysfunctions, sterility (which is reversible), impotence (inability for men to have an erection), prostate enlargement, menstrual irregularities, damage to a developing fetus.

Psychological problems: Depression, listlessness, aggressive and combative behavior.

Other: Acne, edema, hairiness in women, irreversible male pattern baldness in women, oily skin, stunted growth, abdominal pains, chills, diarrhea, changes in bowel and urinary habits, gallstones, hives, headache, excessive calcium, insomnia, kidney stones, kidney disease, muscle cramps, nausea or vomiting, purple or red spots on the body or in the mouth or nose, rash on skin, sore throat, unusual weight gain, unexplained weight loss, unpleasant breath odor, unusual bleeding.

---

should forget about steroids and just work hard, get the proper nutrition, and take sufficient rest. Why attempt to build a strong, healthy muscular system with drugs that are harmful to other body organs, or that might shorten your life?

Increasing Anaerobic Capacity

Anaerobic capacity ("anaerobic" means "without oxygen") is the work done before becoming tired and before oxygen begins to be used in the muscular system. Short bursts of energy like that used in weight lifting and sprinting are examples of the use of anaerobic capacity. Other examples are the short sprints necessary while playing basketball, soccer, hockey, and other such sports.

After the short burst of activity, the muscles need an additional energy source, and so the cells use the food (carbohydrates, proteins, and fats) and the oxygen that is in the blood and is continuously being breathed in. The muscle fibers are now being fueled *aerobically*—with oxygen.

Short-term anaerobic bursts of energy depend on a naturally occurring compound in the body called *creatine*. Creatine is manufactured primarily in the liver, but also in the kidneys and the pancreas. It is essential for muscle functioning as a primary component in the synthesis of *ATP* (adenosine triphosphate), which is used for energy in all cells. When ATP is used up in energy bursts (in about one second), more is resynthesized using the available creatine. But this, in turn, is used up in about five seconds.

While creatine is found in good amounts in both meat and fish, most of it is destroyed in the cooking process. (A normal diet provides about a gram a day.) For this reason, many researchers recommend that serious athletes in power events, or events that require a surge in power, supplement this natural body substance. For these short-term activities, supplementation with *creatine monohydrate* has been found useful to increase the length of time that muscles can work anaerobically. It also aids in developing more force in the muscles so that more weight can be lifted or a sprint start might be faster. (At the time of this writing, the British Olympic medical authorities have taken a position against creatine supplementation for British athletes. It has not, however, been banned by the International Olympic Committee.)

Supplementation is not recommended for the average person; but for the elite-level athlete, it seems to show promise. In a study comparing two groups of strength trainers, one using a placebo and the other creatine, a significant improvement was found for those taking creatine.[1]

Supplementation must be done correctly, however. The recommended dosage is 5 grams of creatine monohydrate four times a day for five days. (Taking more will not help, as the excess is merely excreted in the urine. The tissues can hold only a certain amount.) After this initial high dose, an athlete should take 2 grams a day. After two months, the process is repeated—20 grams a day for five days, then maintaining the level with 2 grams a day. If the muscle storage of creatine had been reduced over the two-month period, it would be brought up to the ideal level by the 20 grams for five days routine.[2]

Fluid and Carbohydrate Replacement

Fluid replacement is essential for people who are sweating because of either their exercise or the outside temperature. The fluid can be replaced along with carbohydrates with a glucose polymer drink. (Glucose polymers are more complex types of sugar than simple sucrose, or table sugar.) Other popular drinks use dextrose or another sugar, along with some of the minerals that are lost in perspiration. Sodium chloride (salt), magnesium, potassium, and calcium are among the common additives to such sport drinks.

While several minerals are lost when one initially sweats, as time passes, the sweat becomes more like pure water. Because of this, pure water is the major need. So if energy replacement is not your objective and cost is a problem, just drink water—lots of it. For some reason, even when we are very thirsty, we generally do not take in as much water as we lose during exercise. You should therefore "force feed" yourself more water.

1 J.S. Volek, et al., "Creatine supplementation enhances muscular performance during high-intensity resistance exercise," *Journal of the American Dietary Association*, July 1997, 97(7), 765–770.

2 We are indebted to Dr. Anna Casey of the Department of Physiology and Pharmacology of the Faculty of Medicine and Health Sciences, The Queen's Medical Centre, Nottingham, England. Dr. Casey is one of the foremost researchers in the world in the area of creatine supplementation.

Fluid-replacement drinks to replace the water and electrolytes lost in perspiration have increased and decreased in popularity recently. First it was thought that only salt and water needed to be replaced after exercise. It was then recognized that other electrolytes (such as potassium) were lost as well, so drinks such as Gatorade became prominent. Later it was recognized that the body tends to conserve its minerals, so athletes were told to drink only water. Now the pendulum has swung once again, and sometimes electrolyte-replacement fluids are recommended.

It has also been learned that simple sugars in the water (as many fluid-replacement drinks contain) retard the absorption of water from the intestines. However, drinks with glucose polymers are absorbed more quickly than plain water. In addition, cool or cold water is absorbed more quickly than warm water.

Shortening the recovery period after exercise by consuming fluids and carbohydrates should be done immediately after a workout or a competition. Whether your workout is a strength-training session or an endurance activity such as running, cycling, or swimming, your maximum recovery cannot occur without an immediate replacement of the carbohydrates lost during the exercise. While many strength trainers think that they need protein replacement, that is incorrect. They need carbohydrates.

International Olympic Committee Medical Code: Prohibited Classes of Substances and Prohibited Methods (January 31, 1997)

I. Prohibited Classes of Substances
  A. Stimulants
  B. Narcotics
  C. Anabolic agents
  D. Diuretics
  E. Peptide and glycoprotein hormones and analogs
II. Prohibited Methods
  A. Blood doping*
  B. Pharmacological, chemical, and physical manipulation
III. Classes of Drugs Subject to Certain Restrictions
  A. Alcohol
  B. Marijuana
  C. Local anesthetics
  D. Corticosteroids
  E. Beta-blockers

*Doping consists of:

1. The administration of substances belonging to prohibited classes of pharmacological agents, and/or
2. The use of various prohibited methods.

Muscle Recovery and Pain Reduction

Anti-inflammatory aids such as aspirin can often reduce muscle soreness, but they also increase one's susceptibility to heat and create a greater risk of heat stroke.

Endurance Enhancement

Stimulants can increase alertness and increase strength and endurance. The only legal stimulant available is *caffeine*. It seems to increase strength by allowing more muscle fibers to be used in a single contraction. It seems to help endurance by increasing the amount of fuel available to the muscles. It does this by allowing the use of the triglyceride blood fats for energy, which thereby preserves the muscle sugars (glycogen) for later in the workout or competition. Caffeine has often been used by runners and cyclists.

Amphetamines and *ephedrine* were once common stimulants, but their use is now prohibited by the athletic community. Even coffee is allowed only up to a certain level by the International Olympic Committee.

Summary

1. Ergogenic aids are whatever facilitate progress toward strength, bulk development, or aerobic or anaerobic work.
2. Ergogenic aids may be legal or illegal substances.
3. To build muscle tissue, a person should take in sufficient amounts of high-quality protein.
4. The use of non-prescription androgenic steroids is illegal and can have serious negative health consequences. Steroids should never be taken as an ergogenic aid.
5. Fluid-replacement drinks can be used to replace the electrolytes and carbohydrates, as well as the fluid, lost through sweat.

13 *Strength-Training Injuries*

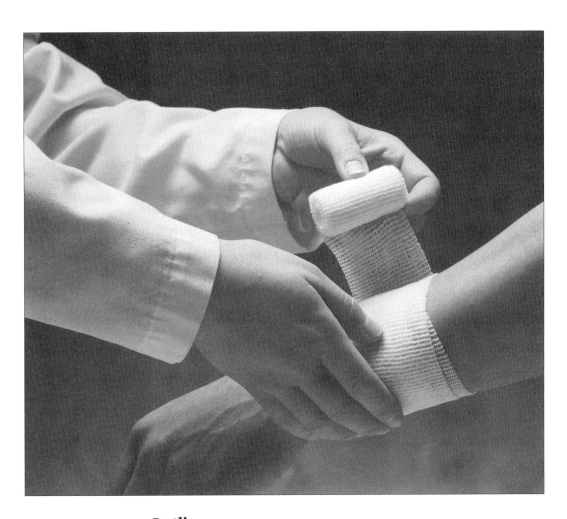

Outline

Strains and Sprains
Back Injuries
Knee Injuries
Arthritis and Joint-Wearing Injuries
High Blood Pressure
Blackouts

Other Injuries
Injury Prevention
Summary

Strength training is a very safe method of training. The reported injury rate for general fitness strength training is about 1.4 injuries per 1,000 participants per year. For more serious bodybuilders (males), it is about 1.4 per 100. The rate for females is even lower—probably because their emphasis tends to be more on technique than on maximum resistance. For Olympic-style lifters, studies indicate a range of injury of between 1.4 and 1.7 per 100, and for power lifters, 1.4 to 3 per 100 participants. Compare this with volleyball's rate of 10 to 50 percent injuries per year, or soccer's 1 injury per 100 hours of participation, and you see that strength training is a very safe activity.

Strains and Sprains

Muscle strains and ligament sprains are the most commonly reported injuries to recreational or school weight trainers. Some of these injuries are very minor and appear only as muscle soreness. Competitive power lifters and Olympic-style lifters are more likely to have a greater degree of muscle or ligament damage because they are lifting much heavier weights. Olympic lifters often have ligament strains in the wrist due to the finishing action of the wrist when bringing the barbell to shoulder level in the clean movement. About 60 percent of the injuries reported by younger power lifters is of the muscular strain variety. However, with more experienced lifters the rate is only about 6 percent for males and 11 percent for females.

Chest (pectoralis major) strains and ruptures are most likely to occur when doing a bench press or supine flys. Be certain to warm up the chest muscles properly before attempting heavy lifting in which they are involved. These ruptures are most likely to happen when the lifter is trying to "max out" on the final repetition.

Shoulder injuries, along with knee problems, are the most common complaint of Olympic lifters. The "clean and jerk" seems to be the most dangerous lift in terms of shoulder injury.

Back Injuries

Low back problems, as might be expected, are common complaints for those lifting heavy weights. The small muscles of the lower back are required to stabilize or move large amounts of weight, particularly in the Olympic lifts and the dead-lift. Spondylolysis (stress fracture of the lower spine) is six times higher among Olympic lifters than the general population (30 percent versus 6 percent). Recreational lifters such as weight trainers need never have this problem. Both bending over to lift the weight from the floor or balancing the weight over the head are problems for Olympic-style lifters.

Power lifters may also suffer low back pain. Two-thirds of power lifters experience such pain at some time, and it is the second most common complaint of female power lifters.

Strengthening of the lower back with the exercises suggested in this book is the best prophylactic against injury. Most serious lifters, however, use weight belts to stabilize the back. Also, orthotic devices in the shoes can properly align the feet and eliminate many problems.

Knee Injuries

Knee injuries among Olympic lifters result from the deep squatting action required for the beginning of the Olympic lifts. More than half of power lifters note similar problems. The knee is the most common source of injuries for female power lifters and female bodybuilders. Weight trainers following the exercises in this book should never have such problems.

Arthritis and Joint-Wearing Injuries

Joint wearing and arthritis are becoming more common with those who do a great deal of lifting. It is the most common complaint of power lifters and body-builders. The continued overuse of the joints may cause tendinitis (inflammation of the tendons), degeneration of cartilage in some joints, and in the advanced stages, arthritis.

High Blood Pressure

High blood pressure at an extremely dangerous level has been recorded in bodybuilders doing some exercises. The normal average blood pressure is 120/80 (enough pressure to move 120 millimeters of mercury when the heart is beating, and 80 millimeters of mercury when the heart is relaxing). A blood pressure of 140/90 is considered too high for safety, and blood-pressure-reducing medicine is usually prescribed. Blood pressures may go as high as 480/350 for some bodybuilders doing double leg presses.

Such high blood pressure can rupture arterioles or arteries in the brain, resulting in a stroke, or arteries in the heart, causing a heart attack. Either a stroke or a heart attack can be major and may result in death, or may be so small that the person doesn't recognize that it has occurred. Even in the latter case, however, some permanent damage can result.

Steroids and improper breathing technique (the Valsalva maneuver) can contribute to high blood pressure.

Blackouts

Blackouts have occurred among lifters who have used the Valsalva maneuver.[1] Strength trainers using the exhaling method of breathing during lifting, as suggested in this book, will not have this problem.

1 D. Compton, P. M. Hill, and J. D. Sinclair, "Weight-lifters' blackout," *Lancet II*, 1973, (7840), 1234–1237.

Other Injuries

Other injuries include finger injuries, which are usually caused when changing weight plates on barbells.

There are few reported injuries of death due to strength training. When it occurs, it is nearly always a male doing a bench press at home and without spotters. Typically the bar falls on the neck or chest, and the lifter dies from suffocation. There are no reported deaths when Olympic lifters, power lifters, or bodybuilders are in competition.

Injury Prevention

Injury prevention is best accomplished by:

- Having a medical clearance (check blood pressure, hernia, poor body alignment)
- Wearing proper clothing (non-skid shoes, hard toes on shoes, absorbent clothing)
- Checking the equipment (tight collars on barbells and dumbbells, no frayed cables on machines, etc.)
- Warming up effectively
- Using the proper technique
- Exhaling while doing the lifting action
- Using spotters in any exercise that might be dangerous or where you might lose your balance

Summary

1. Most sports have some potential for injury, but the rates of injury for strength training are quite low in comparison with other sports.
2. Injuries can often be prevented by proper techniques (including proper breathing), and by effective strengthening of the muscles.
3. Orthotics (shoe inserts) and braces (back, knee, ankle) can greatly reduce the risk of injury.

APPENDIX A

Essential Information on Vitamins and Minerals

Vitamin	Solubility	RDA	Functions	Deficiencies and excesses	Sources
A	Fat soluble Stored in body	5,000 units (men) 1000 Retinol EQ 4,000 units (women) 800 Retinol EQ Toxic level: 25,000 to 50,000 units daily	1. Formation of body tissue. 2. Development of mucous secretions in nose, mouth, digestive tract, organs (which show bacterial entry). 3. Development of visual purple in the retina of the eye, which allows one to see in the dark. 4. Produces the enamel-producing cells of the teeth. 5. Assists normal growth.	Deficiencies can cause: night blindness, damaged intestinal tract, damaged reproductive tract, scaly skin, poor bones, dry mucous membranes, and in children, poor enamel in the teeth. Toxic symptoms (of Retinol): may mimic brain tumor (increased pressure inside the skull), weight loss, irritability, loss of appetite, severe headaches, vomiting, itching, menstrual irregularities, diarrhea, fatigue, skin lesions, bone and joint pains, loss of hair, liver and spleen enlargement, and insomnia. In children, overdose can stunt growth.	Carrots Yellow fruits Green leafy vegetables Butter and margarine Whole milk Liver Fish Fortified nonfat milk Ripe tomatoes Egg yolks
B-1 (thiamin)	Water soluble	1.5 mg (men) 1.1 mg (women)	1. Metabolizes carbohydrates. 2. Resulting glucose (sugar) nourishes muscles and nerves.	Deficiencies can cause: mental depression, moodiness, quarrelsomeness and uncooperativeness, fatigue, irritability, lack of appetite, muscle cramps, constipation, nerve pains (due to degeneration of myelin sheath that covers the nerves), weakness and feeling of heaviness in the legs, beri-beri (a disease in which the muscles atrophy and become paralyzed.	Liver Pork Yeast Organ meats Whole grains Bread Wheat germ Peanuts Milk Eggs Soy beans

Vitamin	Solubility	RDA	Functions	Deficiencies and excesses	Sources
B-2 (riboflavin)	Water soluble	1.8 mg (men) 1.3 mg (women)	Affects rate of growth and metabolic rate since it is necessary for the cell's use of protein, fat, and carbohydrate.	Deficiencies can cause: burning and itching eyes, blurred and dim vision, eyes sensitive to light, inflammation of the lips and tongue, lesions at the edges of the mouth, digestive disturbances, greasy, scaly skin.	Eggs Liver and other organs Yeast Milk Whole grains Bread Wheat germ Green leafy vegetables
Niacin or nicotinic acid	Water soluble Limited storage in the body	20 mg (men) 15 mg (women)	1. Similar to riboflavin in metabolizing foods (especially sugars). 2. Maintains normal skin conditions. 3. Aids in functioning of the gastrointestinal tract.	Deficiencies can cause: Dermatitis (red, tender skin, becoming scaly and ulcerated), fatigue, sore mouth (tongue), diarrhea, vomiting, nervous disturbances, mental depression, anorexia, weight loss, headache, backache, mental confusion, irritability, hallucinations, delusions of persecution, pellagra. Large doses can be toxic because it dilates blood vessels. Can cause skin flushing, dizziness, head throbbing, also dryness of skin, itching, brown skin pigmentation, decreased glucose (sugar) tolerance and perhaps a rise in uric acid in the blood.	Yeast Liver Wheat bran Peanuts Beans
Pantothenic acid	Water soluble Little storage in body	10 mg	1. Carbohydrate, fat and protein metabolism. 2. Synthesis of cholesterol and steroid hormones. 3. Aids the functioning of the adrenal cortex. 4. Aids in choline metabolism.	Almost never deficient in human diets. Various animal studies have shown different results from deficiency: rough skin, diarrhea, anemia, possible coma convulsions, hair loss, and many other symptoms. But they have not been shown in humans.	Liver Organ meats Eggs Yeast Wheat bran Legumes Cereals
Biotin	Water soluble	No RDA	Metabolism of amino acids, fatty acids and carbohydrate.	Deficiencies are extremely rare. Raw egg whites (which combine with the biotin in the intestines and make it unavailable and some antibiotics (which kill the	Manufactured in the intestines Also found in: Liver Yeast Kidney Egg yolks

Vitamin	Solubility	RDA	Functions	Deficiencies and excesses	Sources
				biotin-producing organisms in the intestines) could cause a deficiency. Deficiency would be marked by: dry, scaly skin, gray pallor (skin color) slight anemia, muscular pains, weakness, depression, and loss of appetite.	
B-6 (pyridoxine)	Water soluble	2.0 mg (men) 1.6 mg (women)	Catalyst in protein metabolism. A high-protein diet increases the need for B-6.	Anemia, dizziness, nausea, vomiting, irritability, confusion, kidney stones, skin and mucous membrane problems. In infants: irritability, muscle twitching, convulsion. Excesses: impaired sensation in limbs. Unsteady gait.	Usually not necessary to supplement. Wheat germ Kidney Liver Ham Organ meats Legumes Peanuts
Folic acid (folacin)		200 mcgm (men) 180 mcgm (women)	1. Aids in maturation of red and white blood cells 2. May assist in the synthesis of nucleic acids.	Blood disorders, anemia, diarrhea. Deficiencies most likely to occur during pregnancy and lactation.	Yeast Liver Egg yolk Green leafy vegetables
B-12	Water soluble Stored in the body	2.0 mcgm (men and women)	1. Controls blood-forming defects and nerve involvement in pernicious anemia. 2. Involved in protein, fat, carbohydrate, nucleic acid, and folic acid metabolism. 3. Necessary to the normal functioning of cells, especially in the bone marrow, nervous system, and intestinal tract.	Sore tongue, amenorrhea, signs of degeneration of the spinal cord, anemia, heart and stomach trouble, headache, and fatigue.	Liver Organ meats Oysters Salmon Eggs Beef Milk

Vitamin	Solubility	RDA	Functions	Deficiencies and excesses	Sources
C (ascorbic acid)	Water soluble Little body storage	60 mg (men and women) 10 mg per day prevents scurvy	1. Forms collagen, an intracellular cement that strengthens cell walls (especially the small blood vessels and capillaries), tooth dentine, cartilage, bones, and connective tissue. 2. Aids in the absorption of iron. 3. Aids in formation of red blood cells in the bone marrow. 4. Aids in the metabolism of some amino acids (phenylalanine and tyrosine). 5. May be involved in the synthesis of steroid hormones from cholesterol. 6. Any body stress may deplete the vitamin C in the tissues—shock, fracture, or bacterial infections.	Scurvy results from low vitamin C intake. Minor symptoms of vitamin C deficiency could be: subcutaneous hemorrhages (bleeding below the skin), bleeding from gums, swollen gums Excess of Vitamin C can result in kidney stones and diarrhea, destruction of B-12, acidosis	Citrus Fresh fruits Berries Broccoli Tomatoes Green leafy vegetables Baked potatoes Turnips
D	Stored in liver Fat soluble	10 mcgm	1. Assists in the development of bones and teeth by aiding calcium to harden. 2. Facilitates the absorption of calcium and phosphorus, lack of which can cause muscular cramping.	Deficiencies: ricketts (children), osteomalacia (women who have had frequent pregnancies and poor diets). Teeth may be more susceptible to caries (cavities). Cramping in muscles if there is a low level of calcium or phosphorus in the blood. Soft bones, bowed legs, poor posture. Toxic symptoms: fatigue, weight loss, nausea, vomiting, weakness,	Exposure to ultraviolet light (sunlight) can give minimum daily requirements by changing one type of cholesterol to vitamin D Milk Fish liver oils Egg yolk Butter Whole milk

Vitamin	Solubility	RDA	Functions	Deficiencies and excesses	Sources
				headache, kidney damage, kidney stones, hardening of the soft tissues of the heart, blood vessels, lungs, stomach, and kidneys. Increases cholesterol level of blood. Makes bone more fragile. High levels in developing fetuses and young children may cause mental retardation or blood vessel malformation (especially a blockage in the aorta—the major artery from the heart).	Nonfat milk (with D) Margarines (with D added)
E	Fat soluble (stored in body)	10 mg (men) 8 mg (women)	It is thought to stabilize membranes. May be helpful in stabilizing Vitamin A. Maybe necessary in diets high in polyunsaturated fats, antioxidants.	No known deficiency symptoms in human adults. Some premature infants apparently do not immediately develop the ability to absorb the vitamin.	Synthesized in the intestines. Alpha tocopherol E probably better than mixed-tocopherol E. Human milk (cow's milk poor) Margarine Oil salad dressing Vegetable oils Nuts Eggs Cereal germ Green leafy vegetables
K	Fat soluble	Probably 30–50 mcgm	Helps in the production of prothrombin (blood clotting agent).	Antibiotics taken orally (which could kill the synthesizing bacteria) or diarrhea (which could flush out the bacteria) could possibly cause a deficiency. Newborn infants, especially premature babies, often suffer from a deficiency. This may cause excessive bleeding. Toxic symptoms in infants: jaundice, mild anemia.	Synthesized by intestinal bacteria Green leafy vegetables Cabbage Liver Cauliflower Smaller amounts in: tomatoes, egg yolk and whole milk

Mineral	RDA	Functions	Deficiencies and excesses	Sources
Calcium	1200 mg (men and women)	Development of strong bones and teeth. Help muscles contract and relax normally. Utilization of iron. Normal blood clotting. Maintenance of body neutrality. Normal action of heart muscle.	Rickets, porous bones, bowed legs, stunted growth, slow clotting of blood, poor tooth formation, tetany.	Milk, cheese, mustard, turnip greens, clams, oysters, broccoli, cauliflower, cabbage, molasses, nuts. Small amount in egg, carrot, celery, orange, grapefruit, figs, and bread made with milk
Fluorine	One part per million in water Toxic at 6 to–10 ppm	Resistance to dental caries. Deposition of bone calcium. May be involved in iron absorption.	Deficiencies: weak teeth and bones, anemia, impaired growth. At levels of 1.5 to 4 parts per million teeth will be strong, but may be mottled. At levels over 6 ppm teeth and bones may be deformed.	Water supply containing 1 ppm. Small amount in many foods.
Iodine	0.1 mg (men and women)	Constituent of thyroxine, which is a regulator of metabolism.	Enlarged thyroid gland. Low metabolic rate. Stunted growth. Retarded mental growth.	Iodized salt Sea foods Foods grown in nongoiterous regions
Iron	12 mg (men) 15 mg (women)	Constituent of hemoglobin, which carries oxygen to the tissues.	Nutritional anemia, pallor, weight loss, fatigue, weakness, retarded growth.	Red meats, especially liver, green, vegetables, yellow fruits, prunes, raisins, legumes, whole grain and enriched cereals, molasses, egg yolk, potatoes, oysters
Magnesium	400 mg (men) 300 mg (women)	Activates various enzymes. Assists in breakdown of phosphates and glucose necessary for muscle contractions. Regulates body temperature Assists in synthesizing protein.	Failure to grow, pallor weakness, irritability of nerves and muscles, irregular heartbeat, heart and kidney damage, convulsions and seizures, delirium, depressions.	Soya flour, whole wheat, oatmeal, peas, brown rice, whole corn, beans, nuts

Mineral	RDA	Functions	Deficiencies and excesses	Sources
Phosphorus	800 mg (men & women)	Development of bones and teeth. Multiplication of cells. Activation of some enzymes and vitamins. Maintenance of body neutrality. Participates in carbohydrate metabolism.	Rickets, porous bones, bowed legs, stunted growth, poor tooth formation. Excesses of phosphorus may have same effect on the bones as deficient calcium (osteoporosis-porous bones).	Milk, cheese, meat, egg yolk, fish, nuts, whole grain cereals, legumes, soya flour, whole wheat. oatmeal, peas, brown rice, whole corn, beans
Potassium	2.5 grams	Acid-base balance. Carbohydrate metabolism. Conduction of nerve impulses. Contraction of muscle fibers. May assist in lowering blood pressure (if consumed in equal proportions as sodium).	Apathy, muscular weakness, poor gastrointestinal tone, respiratory muscle failure, tachycardia (irregular heartbeat), cardiac arrest (heart stops beating).	Soybeans, cantaloupe, sweet potato, avocado, raisins, banana, halibut, sole, baked beans, molasses, ham, mushrooms, beef, white potatoes, tomato, kale, radishes, prune juice, nuts and seeds, wheat germ, green leafy vegetables, cocoa, vegetable juices, cream of tartar, prunes, figs, apricots, oranges, grapefruit
Sodium	1-2 grams (1/5 to 2/5 teaspoon)	Constituent of extracellular fluid. Maintenance of body neutrality. Osmotic pressure. Muscle and nerve irritability	Muscle cramps, weakness, headache, nausea, anorexia, vascular collapse. Excess may raise blood pressure.	Sodium chloride (table salt) Sodium bicarbonate (baking soda) Monosodium glutarnate (Accent) The greatest portion of sodium is provided by table salt and salt used in cooking. Foods high in sodium include:

Mineral	RDA	Functions	Deficiencies and excesses	Sources
				Dried beef, ham, canned corned beef, bacon, wheat breads, salted crackers, flaked breakfast cereals, olives, cheese, butter, margarine, sausage, dried fish, canned vegetables, shellfish and salt water fish, raw celery, egg white
Zinc	15 mg (men) 12 mg (women)	Metabolism, formation of nucleic acid.	Impaired growth, sexual development, skin problems.	Beef, chicken, fish, beans

APPENDIX B

Sources of Additional Information (Organizations and Publications)

Organizations

Bodybuilders
International Federation of Body Builders (IFBB)
c/o Weider Enterprises
21100 Erwin Street
Woodland Hills, CA 91367

Conditioning for Athletics
National Strength Conditioning Association (NSCA)
Box 81410
Lincoln, NE 68501

Olympic Weight Lifting
United States Weightlifting Federation (USWF)
U. S. Olympic Complex
1750 E. Boulder Street
Colorado Springs, CO 80909

Power Lifting
Powerlifting U.S.A.
Box 467
Camarillo, CA 93011

National Strength Research Center
Department of Health, Physical Education, and Recreation
2050 Memorial Coliseum
Auburn University, AL 36849

American College of Sports Medicine
Box 1440
Indianapolis, IN 46206

Journals and Magazines

International Weightlifter, Box 65835, Los Angeles, CA 90054

Iron Man, 808 W. Fifth Street, Alliance, NE 69301

National Strength and Conditioning Journal, 251 Capital Beach Blvd., Lincoln, NE 68528

National Strength Research Center Newsletter, Strength-Power Update, 2050 Memorial Coliseum, Auburn University, AL 36849-3501

Sport Fitness, 21100 Erwin Street, Woodland Hills, CA 91367

Strength and Health, Box 1717, York, PA 17405

Strength Training for Beauty, 1400 Stierlin Road, Mountain View, CA 94043

Weightlifters Newsletter, 30 Combria Road, West Newton, MA 02165

World Weightlifting, IWF Secretariat 1374 Budapest, pf 614, Hungary

Reference Books

Baechle, Thomas, ed., *Essentials of Strength Training and Conditioning*, Champaign, IL: Human Kinetics, 1994.

Miller, C. *Olympic Lifting Training Manual*. Iron Man, 808 W. Fifth Street, Alliance, NE 69301

Roman, R. A., and M. S. Shakirzynow. *The Snatch and Clean and Jerk.* Translated by Andrew Chamiga. 11024 Denne, Livonia, MI 48150.

APPENDIX C

Power Lifting: Types of Lifts

1. Bench press
2. Squat
3. Dead-lift (not always in the competition)

Common Weight Classifications

Kilograms	Pounds
52	114.5
56	123.5
60	132.5
67.5	148.75
75	165.25
82.5	181.75
90	198.25
100	220.25
110	242.5
125	275.5
145	318
145+	318+

Possible Divisions in a Tournament

1. Open
2. Novice
3. Drug Free
4. High School
5. Teenage
6. College
7. Masters Age Groups
8. Women

Appendix D

Weight Record Chart

Name	USC Strength														
Date															
Exercise	Reps	Wt.	Reps	Wt.	Reps	Wt.	Reps	Wt.	Reps	Wt.	Reps	Wt.	Reps	Wt.

GLOSSARY

Strength-Training Terms

Abduction   Moving a body segment (an arm or leg) away from the center of the body (such as raising arms from the side to shoulder height).

Adduction   Bringing the body segment back to the center of the body (such as bringing arms back to one's side from an abducted position).

Aerobic   Exercise that requires a great deal of air (oxygen). Such activities as running or swimming for more than 40 seconds are generally in the aerobic category. As the activity progresses, more blood fats and blood sugar (glucose) are used.

Aerobics   A type of cardiovascular exercise. The term is usually associated with a type of aerobic dance routine.

Agonist   The muscle that contracts concentrically, such as the biceps in a curl.

Anabolic steroids   Hormones used to promote muscle growth. They are not recommended and are often illegal.

Anaerobic   Exercise that is completed quickly. Such contractions do not require the presence of oxygen. Lifting heavy weights or running a 100-meter dash are both in the anaerobic category. The fuel for anaerobic activity comes from fuels already in the muscle fibers, not from fats and sugar in the blood.

Antagonist   The muscle opposite the agonist, such as the triceps in a biceps curl.

Barbell   A long steel bar on which weights are attached for two-handed, large-muscle exercises.

Bulk   Increased size of muscle fibers, connective tissues, and "fuel stores." See also hypertrophy.

Cam   Device used in some weight-training machines that aids the lifter in working the muscle to its maximum throughout the contraction. Originated by the developers of the Nautilus machines.

Cardiopulmonary   Means "heart-lungs."

Cardiovascular   Means "heart-blood," but includes the action of the lungs.

Cardiovascular endurance   The body's ability to transport oxygen. It is a reflection of the size and efficiency of the heart, the number of blood vessels carrying oxygen to the muscles, the amount of red blood cells that actually carry the oxygen, and the ability of the muscles to absorb oxygen and utilize it in energy production.

Cardiovascular exercise   Exercise that makes the heart work hard by long-term pumping of blood. (Most experts recommend at least 20 minutes of cardiovascular exercise at your target heart rate.)

Clean and jerk   An Olympic lift in which the bar is brought to chest height in one move (the clean), then brought above the head in a second move (the jerk).

Collars   Metal devices that slide over the end of the bar and hold the weights in place.

Concentric contraction   Occurs when the muscles are shortening.

Curl   An action in which only the elbow or knee joint is moved. It can be a biceps or a leg curl.

Cuts   Term used to define muscle definition in a bodybuilder.

Depression   Downward movement of the shoulders.

Dorsi flexion   Bringing the top of the foot closer to the front of the leg. This action stretches the Achilles tendon.

Dumbbell   Short bar generally used for one-arm exercises.

Eccentric contraction   Occurs when a muscle continues to resist as it lengthens.

Electrolytes   Substances absorbed in solution, capable of conducting electrical charge. The electrolytes calcium, potassium, and magnesium, for example, are essential for nerve and muscle function.

Elevation   Moving the shoulders upward.

Ergogenic   Means "energy producing." Foods and other products that increase energy or speed recovery from fatigue are ergogenic aids.

Eversion   Turning the sole of the foot outward.

Extension   Increasing the angle of a joint (such as letting the bar down to the hips from the chest in a biceps curl).

Flexion   Decreasing the angle of a joint (such as bringing the bar to the chest in a biceps curl).

Hyperextension   Bringing a body part past the normal extension position (such as a back arch).

Hypertrophy   Occurs when the individual muscle fibers increase in size. See also bulk.

Incline-decline board   Padded board that can be set at an angle so that the strength trainer can work different aspects of muscles than those worked in a standing or lying position.

Intensity   The average weight lifted per repetition. It can be seen as the quality of work done in a workout.

Isokinetic   Means "same energy" or "same speed." Refers to exercises performed at a constant rate of speed while force is exerted against a machine. The work done is measured on a gauge. Special machines are required to control the speed of the exercises. The Cybex machine is the most commonly used.

Isometric   Means "same length." The muscle contraction does not change the joint angle.

Isotonic   Means "same tone." Any exercise with free weights.

Inversion   Turning the toe inward.

Lats   Latissimus dorsi muscles of the upper back.

Load   Volume multiplied by the intensity, or the total number of pounds lifted in a workout.

Muscular endurance   Refers to how many contractions a muscle can make without tiring. So it is the ability of the muscle to produce constant force for a long period of time. Running and swimming are examples.

Nautilus   A type of weight machine with special cams that allow adjustment of the amount of force needed to lift the weight so that the muscle can be kept working close to maximum throughout the exercise.

Negative exercise   Eccentric (muscle lengthening) exercise in which the weight is lowered under control to a starting position.

One-repetition maximum (1 RM)   The amount of weight a person can lift one time and one time only.

Periodization   Changing a long-term workout schedule into shorter cycles (periods) during a year.

Plantar flexion   Pushing the toes away from the body (as in a toe raise).

Plyometrics   A rebounding exercise in which the muscle goes immediately from an eccentric to a concentric contraction. It is useful in developing power and speed.

Power   The combination of strength and speed.

Press   An action in which the weight is pushed away from the body using the triceps, shoulder, chest, or leg muscles.

Pronation   Rotating the palm of the hand downward.

Prone   Lying face down.

Repetition   One complete cycle of an exercise (such as raising the bar in a curl, then lowering it).

Rotation   Moving a body part around its long axis (such as moving from pronation to supination or twisting the head).

Set   A number of repetitions performed without resting. Most sets range from three to ten repetitions.

Snatch   Olympic lift in which the weight is lifted from the floor to an overhead position in one movement.

Static contraction   A muscle contraction in which the joint does not move. Isometrics is an example.

Strength   The ability of a muscle group to produce the maximum amount of force. It is shown in how much weight a person can lift one time. It is limited by the number of muscle fibers that can be contracted at one time and by the lever action of a person's joints.

Supination   Rotating the hand upward.

Supine   Lying face up.

Target heart rate   The pulse rate desired by an individual to achieve an effective cardiovascular workout. One popular method is to take 65 to 85 percent of the number that results from subtracting your age from 220.

Ten-repetition maximum (10 RM)   The amount of weight a person can lift ten times but no more.

Universal machines   The first weight machine in which the weights were on slides and were selected by keys.

Valsalva effect   An increase in the pressure inside the chest cavity when the glottis is closed, the breath is held, and the muscles around the chest are contracted. The increased pressure can raise the blood pressure inside the chest significantly.

Volume   The quantity of work done. It is the total number of repetitions done in a workout.

Index

Abdominal exercises, 74-76
Abduction, 26, 100-101
Actin filament, 20
Adduction, 26, 102-103
Aerobic, 8, 17
Aging, effects, 3
Alcohol, 150-151
Amino acids, 133-135, 162
Amphetamines, 167
Anabolic steroids. *See* Steroids
Anaerobic capacity, 164-166
Androgens, 9, 163-164
Angle of exercise, 60
Ankle exercises, 87-91
Ankle sprain, 89
Anorexia nervosa, 156-156
Antagonistic muscular development, 17
Anti-inflammatory drugs, 167
Antioxidants, 139, 163
Archery, 126
Arm exercises, 91-96
Arthritis and strength training, 171
Athletics and weight training, 13, 125-130
    and female athletes, 156
Attire, proper, 3-4, 172

Back arches. *See* Back extensions
Back exercises:
    lower back, 77-79
    upper back, 70-73
Back extensions, 77
Back injuries, 170-171
Badminton players, 126
Balance of muscle strength, 17
Ballistic stretches, 50
Barbells, 183
Baseball players, 126
Basketball players, 126
Bench press, 106-108
Benson, Herbert, 46
Bent flys, 64
Bent row, 116
Beverages, 149-151

Biceps curl, 92
Bioelectrical impedence, 15
Blackouts and Valsalva maneuver, 171
Blood fats, 17
Blood pressure, high, 27, 171
Bodybuilding, 9
    and diet, 132
Body contouring, 13-14
Body fat measurement, 14–15
Body types, 13
Breathing, 27-28
Bulimia, 156-158
Bulk. *See* Hypertrophy

Caffeine, 150, 167
Calf stretch, 54
Calipers, 15
Calories for muscle maintenance, 132-133
Carbohydrates, 8, 137, 162, 165-166
Cardiovascular/cardiorespiratory, 10, 17
    workout for, 34, 129
Chest exercises, 50, 67-70, 124
    for lower chest, 68-70
    for upper chest, 67
Chin-ups, 111
Cholesterol, 17, 136-137, 148-149
Circuit training, 34
Clean, 116
Clean and jerk, 128
Clothing, 3-4, 172
Coffee, 149-150
Cola drinks, 150
Concentration, 46
Concentric contraction, 22, 184
Conditioning, body, 7, 34
Connective tissue, 12
Creatine, 164-165
Curls:
    abdominal, 74-75
    biceps, 92
    leg, 85
Cyclic system, 33, 39
Cyr, Louis, 2

Dead lifts, 77
Decline flys, 70
DeLorme, Thomas, 2
Deltoids, 62-64
Diet, 146-159
Dorsal flexion, 89
Drugs (IOC banned), 166
Dumbbells, 184

Eating disorders, 155-158
Eccentric phase, 9, 22
Ectomorphs, 13-14
Elastic bands, for exercise, 25
Elbow extension, 94
Elbow flexion, 91
Endomorphs, 13-14
Endorphins, 13
Endurance, 6, 8, 10, 167
Ephedrine, 167
Equipment, selecting, 58-60
Ergogenic food and drink, 162-167
Eversion, 89
Examination, medical, 4
Exercise selection, 32, 58
Extension, 26

Fast-twitch fibers, 9, 11, 20-22
Fat, measuring, 14-17
Fats in diet, 135-137
Female athletes, 130, 156
Fiber, dietary, 138
Fibers, muscle, 9, 20-22
Finger injuries, 172
Fitness, 2, 6
Flexibility, 12, 50
   exercises for, 50-56
Flexion, 26
Fluid replacement drinks, 165-166
Focusing, 46
Food additives, 151
Food Guide Pyramid, 146-149
Football players, 126
Forearms, 97
Forward head, 124
Free weights, 23-24

Garfield, Charles, 46-47
Girth measurements, 15-17

Gluteal stretch, 52
Goals, setting, 44, 58
Golfers, 126
Good morning exercise, 78
Groin stretch, 51
Gymnasts, 127

Halteres, 2
Hamstring stretch, 51
Handball players, 127
Hang clean, 118
Height/weight tables, 159
High blood pressure, 27, 171
High pull, 118
Hip abduction, 100-101
Hip adduction, 102-103
Hip extension, 83-85
Hip flexion, 79-81
History of strength training, 2
Home exercise equipment, buying, 25
Hormones, 9-10
Human growth hormone, 9-10
Hydrostatic weighing, 14
Hyperextension, 26
Hyperplasia, 9
Hypertrophy, muscle, 8-9, 10, 12
   diet for, 132
   workout for, 33

Imagery, 45
Incline board, 184
Incline press, 108
Injuries, and strength training, 13, 170-172
Insulin-like growth factors, 9-10
Intensity, 8, 10
Intermediate fibers, 9, 20-22
Inversion, 90
Isokinetic exercises, 23, 25
Isolating joint action, 60
Isolating a muscle, 26, 60
Isometric contractions, 22
Isometric exercises, 23
Isotonic exercises, 23

Joint-wearing injuries, 171

Karvonen formula, 35
Keiser machines, 82

Knee extension, 82-83
Knee flexion, 85-87
Knee injuries, 171

Lat pull-downs, 111-112
Lateral raises. *See* Flys
Latissimus dorsi, 72
Lats stretch, 54
Leg curls, 85
Leg extension, 114
Leg press, 112-115
Lever action, 21
Loading weights, 111
Louganis, Greg, 45
Lower back stretch, 51
Lunge, 115

Machines, 23, 24
Macrocycles, 36
Manual resistance, 25
Medical clearance, 4
Mental benefits, 36, 44
Mental training, 44-47
Mesocycles, 36
Mesomorphs, 13-14
Microcycles, 36
Military press. *See* Standing press
Milk, 146, 148, 149
Milo, 2
Minerals, 139-149, 151, 163, Appendix A
Motivation, 44
Multiple-joint exercises, 106-120
Muscle balance, 17
Muscle bulk, 33-34
Muscle charts, 59
Muscle contractions, types of, 22-23
Muscle fibers, 9, 20-22
Muscle hypertrophy, 8-9, 10, 12, 20, 33, 132
Muscle size, 9
Muscles:
    building, 33-34, 162
    isolating, 26
    recovery of, 167
    soreness of, 29
Muscular endurance, 6, 8, 10, 167
Myosin, 20

National Strength and Conditioning Association, 177
Nautilus machines, 23
Neck exercises, 60-62
Nicklaus, Jack, 45
Nutrition, 132-143, 162-163

Olympic lifts, 2, 119, 128
One repetition maximum (1 RM), 7
Order of exercises, 32
Organizations, 177
Overeating, 152-153
Overhead barbell press, 108-111

Periodization, 36, 40
Phytochemicals, 141-142
Plantar flexion, 185
Plyometrics, 11-12, 185
Positions, 26
Posture, 12-13, 122-125
Pot belly, 13, 122-123
Power, 11, 12, 185
Power clean, 116-118
Power lifting, 2, 9, Appendix C
Power snatch, 118-119
Preservatives in food, 151
Press, 185
Priority system, 32-33, 39
Progressive resistant exercise, 2
Pronation, 26, 185
Prone, 186
Protein, 9, 133
Pullovers, 73
Pulse rate, 34
Pyramid system, 33, 39

Racquetball players, 127
Recording progress, 37-40, Appendix D
Rehabilitation, 2, 13
Rehearsal, mental, 47
Relaxation, 46
Repetitions, 7-8, 10, 12, Appendix D
Resistance training, 9-10, 23-26
Rest, 36
Reverse pyramid system, 33, 39
Rotator cuff exercises, 65-67

Round shoulders, 123
Rowing, bent, 116
Rowing, upright, 115

Salt, 151
Seated shoulder stretch, 50
Sets, 7, 186
  rest between, 36
Sex differences, 8
Shoulder exercises, 13, 50, 62-64, 71, 123
Shoulder press. *See* Standing press
Shoulder rotation, 50
Shoulder stretch, 123
Shrugs, 71
Side sit-ups, 75-76
Single-joint exercises, 58-103
Skiers, 70, 127
Slow-twitch fibers, 9, 20-22
Snatch, 118
Soccer players, 127
Softball players, 126, 127
Soreness, 29
Specificity of training, 11
Speed, 11
Split routines, 34, 39
Sprains, 170
Springs, for exercise, 25
Squat rack, 112-113
Squats, 112-115
Standing press, 108-109
Static contractions, 22
Static stretch, 50
Steroids, 9, 163-164
Stimulants, 167
Strains, 170
Strength training:
  body positions for, 26
  developing, 7, 32
  injuries and, 13, 170-172
  mental benefits of, 44-45
  planning program for, 6-7, 32-41
  reasons for, 2-3, 6
  resources for, Appendix B
Stretching, 50-56
Sugar, 151
Super sets, 34, 40
Supination, 26, 186
Supine fly, 68

Supplements:
  creatine, 164-165
  protein, 134
  vitamins and minerals, 162-163, Appendix A
Swimming, 70, 94, 127-128

Target heart rate, 34, 35
Tea, 150
Ten repetition maximum (10 RM), 7
Tennis players, 128
Testosterone, 9-10
Thigh and groin stretch, 53-54
Track and field, 128
Trapezius, 72
Triceps stretch, 54
Triglycerides, 17
Trunk twist, 52-53

Universal Gym, 23-24
Upright row, 115-116
USRDA, 133

Valsalva maneuver, 27, 171
Vegetarianism, 151
Visualization, 45
Vitamins, 138-139, 151, 163, Appendix A
Volleyball players, 128
Volume, 8, 186

Warm-up, 28-29
  and stretching, 55
Water, 142, 165
Weight/height tables, 159
Weight lifting, 129
Weight loss, 152-155
Weight machines, 23-24
Weight record chart, Appendix D
Workouts:
  for general conditioning, 34
  for muscle bulk, 33-34
  progression of, 32, 56
  recording progress, 37-40, Appendix D
  rest between, 36
  schedule for, 32-41
  for specific sports, 125-129
  for strength, 32, 125-129
Wrestling, 129
Wrist exercises, 97-100